"*Real Food All Year* puts the joy back into eating seasonally. A food educator with a background in Chinese medicine, Nishanga Bliss has meticulously researched how the seasons affect our bodies and gives lively instructions for enriching our connection to spring, summer, winter, and fall through mindful eating. Her recipes fuse fine dining with traditional hippie food to create astoundingly tasty dishes like kale caesar salad and red lentil dal with sweet corn. As a gardener, I found the book a delight: a pat on the back that endorses growing your own food and also a gentle reminder to harvest my root vegetables so I can make a batch of pickled beets and turnips."

> —Novella Carpenter, author of *Farm City* and *The Essential Urban Farmer*

"This is an excellent and intriguing book. Its overview of the seasons is quite comprehensive, the recipes are really well chosen and easy to make, and there is a lot of excellent scientific information in the text. This would be a worthwhile addition to any health-oriented cook's collection!"

> —Annemarie Colbin, PhD, founder and CEO of the Natural Gourmet Institute in New York City and author of *The Whole-Food Guide to Strong Bones*

"Deftly weaving together the principles of seasonality, sustainability, and healthy eating from a Chinese medicine perspective, Nishanga Bliss does something entirely new—she presents a system for eating that is both sensible and meaningful. *Real Food all Year* is a fascinating and inspiring read that goes far beyond the usual gastronomic reasons for eating local foods in season, but isn't afraid to fully celebrate the pleasures of the table. Call it hedonism Rx."

> —Vanessa Barrington, author of *DIY Delicious*

"*Real Food All Year* is filled with invaluable tips and sound advice. Follow the guidance in this book and find yourself coming back into balance both in your health and with the natural world that surrounds you."

—Margaret Floyd, NTP, HHC, CHFS, author of *Eat Naked* and *The Naked Foods Cookbook*

"*Real Food All Year* is filled with important practical information on nutrition and seasonality. Author Nishanga Bliss clearly explains essential concepts from both Chinese medicine and Western nutritional science and applies them with mouth-watering recipes and easy-to-follow techniques. This book is a valuable resource for anyone seeking to find their way back to the simplicity and harmony of local, seasonal eating."

—Sandor Ellix Katz, author of *Wild Fermentation, The Revolution Will Not Be Microwaved,* and *The Art of Fermentation*

"I've been waiting for a book like this for years! Nishanga Bliss makes the ancient wisdom of traditional Chinese medicine accessible and relevant to today's readers. She deftly weaves these time-tested teachings together with a practical approach to eating locally, seasonally, and sustainably. Well-written and full of useful information and recipes, this will book will be a resource I turn to again and again."

—Jessica Prentice, owner of Three Stone Hearth Community Supported Kitchen

"I am a big fan of eating locally and seasonally as a vital part of healthy nutrition. Nishanga Bliss has created this wonderful new book, *Real Food All Year,* that helps us enjoy her great guidance and sumptuous recipes."

—Elson M. Haas, MD, integrated medicine practitioner and author of *Staying Healthy with the Seasons*

real food all year

Eating
Seasonal
Whole Foods
for
Optimal Health &
All-Day Energy

Nishanga Bliss, MSTCM, LAc

New Harbinger Publications, Inc.

Publisher's Note

This publication is designed to provide accurate and authoritative information in regard to the subject matter covered. It is sold with the understanding that the publisher is not engaged in rendering psychological, financial, legal, or other professional services. If expert assistance or counseling is needed, the services of a competent professional should be sought.

Distributed in Canada by Raincoast Books

Copyright © 2012 by Nishanga Bliss
New Harbinger Publications, Inc.
5674 Shattuck Avenue
Oakland, CA 94609
www.newharbinger.com

Hibiscus and Rose Hip Soda recipe adapted from FULL MOON FEAST by Jessica Prentice, copyright © 2006. Used by permission of Chelsea Green Publishing. www.chelseagreen.com

Cover design by Amy Shoup; Interior art by Sheila Metcalf-Tobin; Acquired by Melissa Kirk; Edited by Clancy Drake

Library of Congress Cataloging-in-Publication Data

Bliss, Nishanga.
  Real food all year : eating seasonal whole foods for optimal health and all-day energy / Nishanga Bliss ; Foreword by Liz Lipski.
    p. cm.
  Includes bibliographical references.
  ISBN 978-1-60882-155-6 (pbk.) -- ISBN 978-1-60882-156-3 (pdf e-book) -- ISBN 978-1-60882-157-0 (epub)
  1. Cooking (Natural foods) 2. Food supply--Seasonal variations. 3. Diet therapy. 4. Cookbooks. I. Title.
  TX741.B578 2012
  641.3'02--dc23

                               2011044395

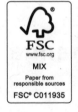

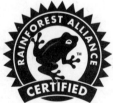

Printed in the United States of America

14   13   12

10   9   8   7   6   5   4   3   2   1   First printing

To my grandmothers, and to grandmothers everywhere.

Contents

Foreword

Nishanga Bliss wants us to incorporate more traditional foods into our diet. *Real Food All Year*, with its delectable descriptions of food, markets, and cooking techniques, will seduce you into wanting to shop, cook, and possibly even grow your own food—and you'll be convinced by science that is relevant to our daily lives and health.

Over millennia, cultures developed agricultural methods, cooking, and eating in harmony with other people and with the seasons. There was a lot of trial and error involved in discovering which foods worked to enhance health and well-being. In all cultures, food was prepared (whether soaked, cooked, sprouted, pounded, or fermented) in ways that ensured optimal digestion and absorption. People prepared and ate food in groups. There was a connection with community, season, and place.

In our culture, all of this has changed. Modern agriculture has separated us from the food we eat so that we don't really know where our food comes from. We eat different types of foods than our ancestors ate. According to government surveys, many of us fail to regularly get the recommended dietary allowances of many nutrients. We eat on the run, we eat by ourselves, and we eat food that is generally nutrient depleted and inflammatory. We eat what's fast, easy, and convenient. Forty-five percent of our meals are eaten away from home. More than a quarter of us get over a third of our calories each day at fast food restaurants. This typical

Western diet is inflammatory, and inflammation underlies virtually all illness. In a few short generations, we've gone from a culture that had basically no cancer, diabetes, or heart disease to a culture that is riddled with these diseases. As societies move to a more processed, westernized way of eating, chronic disease appears. When I first began working as a nutritionist thirty years ago, one person in eight developed cancer in the United States; now half of all men and one-third of all women will develop cancer. When people return to eating more "real food" prepared in traditional ways, incidence of disease goes down.

Food is more than just nutrients. It's information for your genes and your cells. The new field of nutritional genomics informs us that each time we eat, the food sends signals to our genes and cells telling them what to do. When we eat a dinner of broiled fish, steamed greens, and brown rice, our response is different than when we eat, let's say, a fast food meal or a frosted cappuccino mocha.

This book brings us back to our cultural traditions and invites us to embrace our food more fully. Nishanga Bliss synthesizes Chinese wisdom and current Western scientific information about food and puts it into a context that is practical and engaging. Her intimate knowledge and personal writing style hold our attention. She offers a detailed step-by-step guide with shopping lists, recipes, and even recommendations about which cooking utensils to use. We can renew ourselves in spring with detoxifying greens and omega-3–rich lamb koftas. We can spend our summers cooling off with probiotic-laden hibiscus and rose hip soda. In autumn we can ground ourselves with roasted root vegetables, or white bean and kabocha squash stew with herbed pesto. In winter we can alkalinize and renew our digestive system and bones with hearty homemade broths and soups. Enticing, to be sure. This book takes us on a trip through the seasons where we delight to find out more about our own rhythms and how to eat to nourish our body and spirit.

—Elizabeth Lipski, PhD, CCN, CHN
Education Director and Director of Doctoral Studies
Hawthorn University
Author of *Digestive Wellness and Digestive Wellness for Children*

Acknowledgments

A big thank you to all the wonderful folks at New Harbinger for helping me make this book a reality. I am grateful to my many teachers, and to my clients and students—I continue to learn from you each day. Many thanks to my loved ones who gave me the space and support I needed to write.

Introduction

We Americans are eating ourselves to death. According to the Centers for Disease Control, the top three causes of death in the United States are linked to poor diet and inactivity. This generation of American children can expect shorter life spans than their parents, due largely to the sad effects of the standard American diet (Olshansky et al. 2005). If you've picked up this book, you probably already have a sense that something is out of balance: your health or energy levels might be less than optimal, you might be eating healthfully but feel there is more that you can do, you might be concerned with the state of the food system, or you may simply be seeking inspiration in the kitchen. This book offers fresh answers to the age-old question of what to eat?

In 2009, the average American supermarket carried almost fifty thousand products, according to the national Food Marketing Institute. Consider what guides your food choices when you are out shopping. Is it habit? Tradition? Taste? Pleasure? Advertising? Product placement? Science? Health concerns? Sustainability? There is so much conflicting information about what to eat today that negotiating the vast number of choices in the modern marketplace can be overwhelming. *Real Food All Year* offers a unique perspective to guide you: it integrates contemporary nutrition research with the ancient teachings of Chinese medicine to help you create a way of cooking and eating that is seasonal, sustainable, and appropriate for your body, and that can lead you to optimal energy and health. This book offers an adaptation of traditional dietary wisdom to the food supply and health concerns of contemporary North Americans.

Why Chinese Medicine?

You might wonder what makes the insights of Chinese medicine on nutrition so relevant to our times. Chinese medicine is one of the most widely used traditional health systems on the planet. The texts on which it is based were written over two thousand years ago and are thought to represent a compilation of thousands of years of observation and clinical practice before that (Ho and Lisowski 1997). While human lives have changed radically since that time, human physiology has in fact changed very little. The effectiveness of Chinese medicine has been continually validated as its practice has flourished and spread across the globe, and many of its insights are being confirmed by modern scientific research; these convergences will be highlighted throughout this book.

Chinese medicine offers an important complement, and counterpoint, to Western allopathic medicine in that, like most other non-Western medicines, it is truly *holistic*, meaning that it is concerned with "the complete psychological and physiological individual" (Kaptchuk 2000, 4). Health in the Chinese medical system is seen as a state of balance, or harmony, between opposing forces, which can be couched in contemporary physiological terms as a state of dynamic equilibrium, or *homeostasis*, both within an individual and between an individual and her or his environment. The goal of vibrant health, or vitality, includes not only resistance to disease or but also appropriate energy levels, emotional balance, and longevity. A key way to reach this goal is through the diet.

Balancing Your Diet

While your grandmother and your nutritionist might both advise you to eat a balanced diet, they may mean two very different things by "balance."

A Western science–based conception of a balanced diet usually refers to eating a mix of food groups, or *macronutrient* (protein, carbohydrate, and fat) types. By contrast, traditional Asian nutrition, embedded in culture and folk wisdom, categorizes foods according to their *energetic* qualities, providing a way of summarizing the effects of ingesting foods on the body. The simplest system is based on a fundamental concept in Asian medicine, culture, and philosophy: the division between *yin* and *yang*. All phenomena are divided into one of these two major categories, which are both oppositional and interdependent, for example:

Yin	Yang
Dark	Light
Wet	Dry
Water	Fire
Night	Day
Reduced activity	Hyperactivity
Body structures	Physiological functions

Foods are categorized as either *warming* (yang) or *cooling* (yin). Warming foods tend to provide more thermal energy and macronutrient calories, while cooling foods tend to be less calorie dense, instead having higher water content and being relatively rich in micronutrients. Warming foods tend to stimulate or speed up metabolic processes, while cooling foods tend to slow them down and also to exert anti-inflammatory effects. Health requires an ever-shifting balance of the two. In general, animal-flesh foods, alcohol, and certain hot spices are considered more warming, while dairy, eggs, beans, and grains are neutral in energy, and most other plant foods, such as fruits and vegetables, are cooling to the body. Within these larger categories of foods, individual foods are characterized as relatively more yin or yang. For example, plant foods that grow below ground, such as root vegetables, as well as those that take longer to grow, are generally more warming than those that grow above ground or grow more quickly, like leafy greens. Foods of warmer colors, such as red, orange, or yellow, are generally more warming than foods of cooler colors, such as blue, green, purple, or black. Produce from tropical climates is generally much more cooling than that from temperate climates.

Eat with the Seasons

As you proceed through the book, you will learn that in-season foods tend to complement the prevailing season, helping our bodies adjust to the climate, supporting health, and preventing the illnesses typical of that time of year. Cooling vegetables, such as cucumbers and summer squash, ripen in the summertime and, when eaten then, help to cool the body and provide fluids and extra antioxidants needed when we are exposed to more sunshine. By contrast, vegetables that mature in winter, such as kale and broccoli, and those that store well to last throughout the year, like onions and winter squash, are more warming, typically providing more calories and a different set of beneficial phytonutrients.

Just as important as the energy of the food itself is the effect of the method of preparing it. Intuitive cooks and worldwide culinary traditions make use of this principle all the time. Imagine eating a salad of raw shredded carrots, dressed with lemon juice and olive oil. Would that sound good on a hot day? Now imagine the very different effect of eating those carrots if you roasted them in olive oil, allowing the sugars to caramelize, and then drizzled them with the lemon juice. Such a dish would be much more hearty and satisfying in cold weather, right? Cooking methods in order from warming to cooling are: deep frying, roasting, baking, sautéing, pressure cooking, simmering, steaming, fermenting, marinating, sprouting, and serving raw. You'll learn to use these different methods to prepare meals appropriate for the season and your state of health.

There are many benefits to be gleaned from eating according to the seasons. From the point of view of Western nutrition, in-season food simply contains more nutrients. For example, in a 2008 study evaluating the vitamin C content of supermarket broccoli, a research team found that locally harvested fall broccoli had almost twice the vitamin C content of imported spring broccoli (Wunderlich et al. 2008), which had traveled many miles to reach the market. Since produce tends to lose nutrients after harvest, the shorter the time from harvest to your plate, the more nutritious your food will be. For example, in a 2004 study at Penn State, Luke LaBorde and his team found that spinach lost 47 percent of its folate by seven days after harvest (Pandrangi and LaBorde 2004).

Remember the adage of both grandmothers and nutritionists to "eat a variety of foods"? As an added bonus to the sheer pleasure of this style of eating, varying your diet according to the seasons increases the variety of the food you eat, which in itself is associated with improved nutrition and resistance to chronic disease (Tucker 2001).

The Theory of the Five Elements

Chinese medicine and other Asian health systems, such as the macrobiotic diet, a contemporary adaptation that focuses on eating whole grains and vegetables and avoiding processed or refined foods, draw on the ancient theory of the five elements. This theory appears in the most influential ancient text of Chinese medicine, *The Yellow Emperor's Classic of Medicine*, or *Nei Jing*, written as early as 300 BCE (Ni 1995). Five element theory is based on the close observation of the natural world, and it permeates not only the cuisines but also the literature, art, and belief systems of Asian cultures. The five element cycle describes the changes of seasons and the way that living things are born, grow, flourish, wither, and die in repeating patterns. As you get to know this system, you will be able to observe many examples of these cyclical changes in your life and in the world around you. Attention to the cycle can guide you on a path to wellness and remind you of the healthiest ways to live and eat throughout the year. Each element corresponds to a particular season of the year and to a major internal organ. The five elements are often portrayed as a seasonal cycle, as follows:

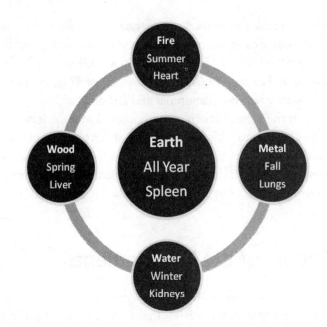

To understand and use this system, it is important to grasp some of the differences between Chinese and Western medicine. As you study the above chart, remember that the traditional Chinese understanding of the body organs is quite different from that of Western physiology. It evolved primarily from clinical observation, not dissection. The organs in this system are best thought of as representing not only the physical internal organs but also the entire body system of which they are a part. For example, the spleen in Chinese medicine is the primary organ of digestion, and may be thought of as encompassing the functions of the spleen, stomach, pancreas, and other parts of the digestive tract as it is understood in Western medicine. In all, this is thought of as the *energy* of the spleen. Note that spleen weakness in the Chinese medicine sense does not necessarily indicate any disorder of the spleen organ in the Western medical sense but instead indicates less than optimal digestive function. As I discuss each season throughout the book, I will explain how Chinese medicine views the related organs, as well as the corresponding thinking in Western medicine.

There are five primary internal organs: the heart, spleen, lungs, kidneys, and liver, and each is paired with one or more secondary organs; for example, the stomach is paired with the spleen and the gallbladder with the liver. The internal organs are seen to work synergistically to create the physiological functions of the body. Imbalances in each organ can lead to symptoms and ill health. These imbalances generally fall into one of two types: *excess*, characterized by hyper function, acute inflammation, and/or congested energy or blood flow; and *deficiency*, which may entail reduced function, chronic inflammation, structural damage, and/or reduced energy or blood flow.

If you've visited a practitioner of Chinese medicine or related arts, you may have been diagnosed, for example, with *liver qi congestion*, one of the most common imbalances among North Americans (*qi* means, essentially, energy). This diagnosis describes a pattern of disharmony or less-than-optimal function, not literally of your liver organ but of the physiological system to which it is connected. Each pattern of excess or deficiency in a particular organ is associated with a characteristic set of signs and symptoms.

The *Nei Jing* teaches that each of the five elements corresponds to one of the major internal organ systems as well as to a particular season. It is beneficial to attend to the health of each organ in its corresponding season. While an imbalance or illness can affect an organ during any season, many health problems can be treated or, better yet, prevented by adjusting the diet—making it more warming or cooling—and by choosing foods to either strengthen or cleanse a particular organ. Following the wheel of the year and echoing the rhythms of nature by choosing seasonal food and preparing it appropriately will ensure that each organ and system is strengthened and cleansed in turn, promoting balanced energy and vitality. The *Nei Jing* also teaches that it is normal for our energy levels to change throughout the year. Summer, for example, is considered the time of maximum energy and activity levels, while in winter we are advised to go to bed early and rise with the sun, focusing on conserving energy and replenishing ourselves.

Real Benefits from Real Food

These ancient Chinese medical concepts of the effects of food are based on *real food*, that is, fresh, whole food that has been grown or produced with minimal refining and without chemical inputs. Unfortunately, much food eaten in North America today is not real food. Most of our choices are, in the words of best-selling author Michael Pollan (2008, 1), "edible foodlike substances…highly processed concoctions designed by food scientists, consisting mostly of ingredients derived from corn and soy." To reap the health benefits of eating properly, we need to return to eating (mostly) real food. This doesn't have to be 100 percent of the time—wise grandmothers and nutritionists know that striving for complete dietary compliance is foolish. Strive to eat as well and as consciously as you can 80 percent of the time and allow yourself to eat whatever you feel like the rest of the time. As your palate adjusts to the subtler flavors of real food prepared consciously, the desire for many refined foods often simply fades away.

Finding Real Food

One way to recognize real food is that it is whole. Whole food includes whole grains, whole fruits and vegetables, and whole animals. Eating whole fruit, for example, offers a much wider range of nutrients than drinking fruit juice. When grains are milled and refined, vitamins, minerals, and fiber are lost. This principle holds true for animal foods as well. Traditional peoples prized the parts of animals often neglected today, such as the organs, glands, and bones, for their concentrated nutrition. In general, eating whole foods best supports health. That said, all processing of food is not bad. While industrial processing and refining of foods generally decreases their nutritional value and adds potentially harmful compounds such as preservatives and additives, most traditional methods of food processing, like soaking, fermentation, and sprouting, actually increase the nutritional value and digestibility of food (Lipski 2010). You'll learn many of these techniques in subsequent chapters.

Real food can be found at the supermarket. It is hidden in plain sight around the perimeter, in the produce, meat, and dairy cases, and perhaps the bulk bins. Follow these two rules when shopping at the supermarket: look for food that has no label because it does not come in a box, bag, or package; and if it does have a label, avoid it if it has more than five ingredients or contains ingredients that you would never use when cooking in your own kitchen (Pollan 2008). Shopping at natural food stores makes this easier, but you still need to be wary. There are many "natural" products on the shelves that are still highly refined. When you shop at one of the thousands of farmers' markets across the nation, you can feel confident that you are choosing real food. Plus, you get to connect with the people growing your food and with your community. Sociologists have found that farmers' market shoppers have ten times more conversations while shopping than supermarket shoppers (Halweil 2004). See Resources if you need help finding a farmers' market in your area.

Community supported agriculture (CSA) is another wonderful resource for accessing real food from the source. The basic model is this: you subscribe (typically for a week, month, or year) to the products of a farm, paying the farmer directly and in advance. You pick up your produce from a nearby drop-off point, or for an extra fee, some farms will deliver to you. The benefits are many: by eliminating the middleman, the farmer gets a better price (which can enable small family farms to compete in the marketplace), you get to connect with the source of your food, and you receive the freshest and most delicious produce imaginable, in season. You also get exposed to wonderful new foods you might have never eaten otherwise, and most CSAs offer a newsletter or other resources to teach you how to cook any unfamiliar produce. There are CSAs for fruits and vegetables, grains and beans, meat and dairy, and even honey (see the resources section).

Produce sold at farmers' markets, farm stands, and CSAs is much more likely to have been harvested when ripe because of the shorter time it takes to get to you. Fruits and vegetables allowed to ripen on the plant taste better, and most are more nutritious than their counterparts, which are commonly harvested earlier and ripened artificially (Lee 2000). An additional nutrition bonus of food from the small family farms that typically sell to farmers' markets and CSAs is the diversity of species they grow. Industrial-scale farms usually select varietals based on uniformity and yield, which has been shown to result in lowered nutritional value (Davis et al. 2004), while smaller-scale farmers often grow more diverse and heirloom varietals, which can pack a higher nutritional and flavor punch. Finally, organically grown plant foods have been shown, in a recent meta-analysis of every peer-reviewed study published since 1980 on the topic, to be nutritionally superior to food grown by conventional methods. On average, according to the research team at The Organic Center, a "serving of organic plant-based food contains about 25% more of the [11] nutrients encompassed in this study than a comparable-sized serving of the same food produced by conventional farming methods" (Benbrook 2008). The nutritional superiority of food produced organically largely derives from the rich soil that organic practices such as composting create, as well as the strict limitation of chemical inputs that organic certification mandates.

The finest nutrition of all can be obtained from foods you grow, sprout, forage, or raise yourself. The gardener's delight of eating straight out of the garden provides superb nutrition, is deeply seasonal, and is accessible, through sprouting, to all (see chapter 2). Foraging and gleaning in your neighborhood or wild places adds a whole new repertoire of seasonal delights to your diet. Finally, beekeeping, backyard poultry and goats, and other endeavors in homesteading can reconnect you to seasonal rhythms and turn you from a consumer to a producer of real food. The Resources section has books and websites to inspire you to get started.

What about Animal Products?

Animal foods are an important part of the diet for most people, yet many of us have concerns about the safety, sustainability, and source of animal foods. A basic rule of thumb when choosing animal products is, from the pen of Michael Pollan (2008, 167), "you are what what you eat eats too." In short, the better the diet and life of an animal, the more nutritious are its meat, milk, or eggs (Robinson 2004). While factory-farmed animal products can have greater negative health and environmental impacts than almost any other food in your diet, choosing animal foods from sustainable sources is one of the most powerful ways you can positively influence your health and the food system. Seeking out organic or, better yet, pasture-raised animal products will have a big impact on your health and that of the planet, and will help support sustainable animal husbandry. You'll read more about the benefits of pasture-raised animal foods in chapter 2.

In general, as with other animal food, the better a fish's diet, the more nutritious it is. Wild trumps farmed in most cases. Many farmed fish have been found to contain contaminants and industrial pollutants, and they are often fed a very poor diet. However, the world's fish stocks are in imminent danger of collapse from overfishing and environmental destruction. Fish may be a healthy choice for us as individuals in the short run, but choosing fish from a fishery on the verge of collapse can't be a healthy choice for us, collectively, in the long run. The conscientious fish eater must continuously learn about the sources of fish. Because the state of the world's fish stocks is changing so quickly, Internet-based resources may be the most accurate. Try www.thefishlist.org, created by three reputable research and scientific bodies, for up-to-date information on both the state of fisheries and the health risks of certain kinds of fish and seafood.

What if you choose to avoid animal foods for religious, spiritual, or political reasons? Chinese medicine has traditionally emphasized the importance of an omnivorous diet as the best for health. Recall the categorization of foods into those with warming or cooling energies. Animal foods are generally warming, while plant foods are much more cooling. Chinese doctors observe that many who go on extended vegetarian and vegan diets eventually exhibit signs of *coldness* and/or digestive weakness, with such complaints as bloating after meals, fatigue, feeling cold, and more. Those who choose to limit or avoid animal foods can improve their health by shifting the diet to make it more warming and cooking and eating in ways that are strengthening to digestion, following the principles described in this book. They may also use the recipes in this book to begin introducing the most beneficial animal foods, such as animal fats and bone broth, to create a diet that will support their health long term. Many of the recipes in this book can be adapted for those who limit animal foods in the diet, for example, by substituting tamari for fish sauce and vegetable stock for bone broth.

The profound benefits of attuning your diet to the seasons go beyond personal health. Cooking and eating seasonally brings you into harmony with natural cycles, connects you to ancient human traditions almost forgotten in the modern era, teaches that personal and planetary health are interdependent, and can become a source of tremendous pleasure and satisfaction in your life.

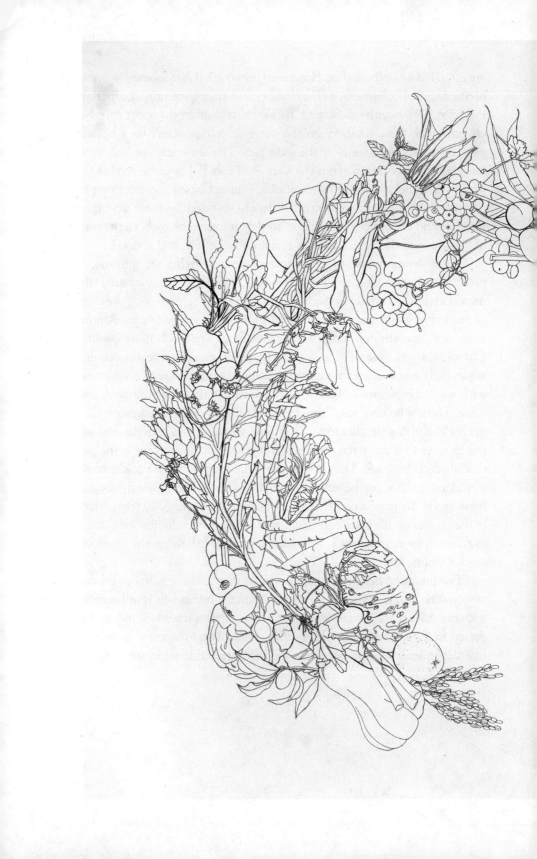

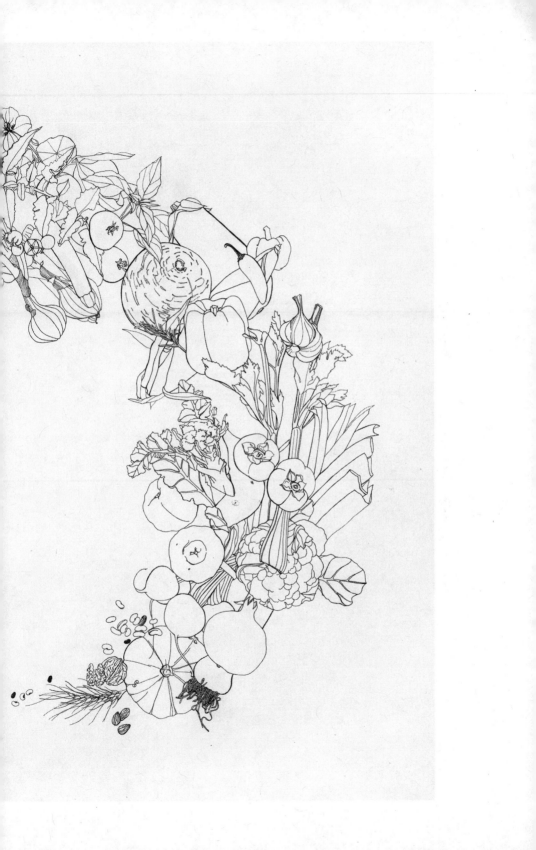

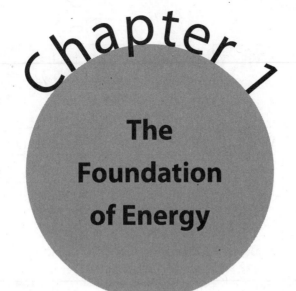

Chapter 1

The Foundation of Energy

Until the last hundred years or so, human lives and diets have been closely tied to the rhythms of the seasons. The advent of industrial agriculture and food technology, along with the increasing role of imported food from distant climates, has changed that—to the detriment of human and planetary health. To return to a wiser way of eating and living, we will examine the wisdom of the ancients, as well as of our grandmothers. Local, seasonal food, prepared and eaten properly, naturally supports vibrant health and energy.

Remember the theory of the five elements? Each element corresponds to a season, a taste, a set of internal organs, a color, one or more stages of plant growth, certain foods, and more. The wood element, for example, represents the dominant energy of springtime, the liver and gallbladder organs, the sour taste, the color green, and the emotion of anger. For optimal wellness, you should attend to the health of each internal organ during its corresponding season. The following table lists some basic correspondences, which will be explored through the rest of the book.

Season	Spring	Summer	Late Summer/ Year- Round	Fall	Winter
Element	Wood	Fire	Earth	Metal	Water
Organ	Liver	Heart	Spleen	Lung	Kidney
Taste	Sour	Bitter	Sweet	Pungent*	Salty
Color	Green	Red	Yellow	White	Black
Stage of Plant Growth	Sprouts, shoots, and leaves	Flowers, early fruits	(not applicable)	Mature fruits and root crops	Seeds
Animal Food	Poultry, eggs, and dairy	Lamb	Beef	Traditional: horse Modern: fish	Pork
Grain	Wheat, rye	Corn, quinoa	Millet	Rice	Beans
Emotion	Anger	Joy	Worry	Grief	Fear

You may be surprised to see five seasons instead of four in the chart above. In the Chinese system, there is a fifth season, known as late summer. The earth element is associated with the season of late summer, and it also occurs throughout the year. Earth is often portrayed as the center of the wheel of the year, linking earth to the energy of harmony, or balance, between yin and yang, which is important for health year-round. The association of earth with the spleen, and indeed the digestive system as a whole, underscores the importance of digestion in Chinese medicine. The classic texts of Chinese medicine explain that spleen qi and stomach qi are

* Spicy but not necessarily hot

the root of a person (Maciocia 1989). Strong digestive energy is linked to good health, long life, and a good prognosis in the case of disease.

Maximum Digestion, Maximum Energy

Our exploration of how to eat seasonally for optimal health and energy must begin with an exploration of digestion, as this is the means by which our bodies extract energy from the food we eat. Looking at the digestive system first from the perspective of traditional Asian medicine and then through the lens of contemporary Western medical science will yield insights from both systems that will help you get the most energy and nutrition from your food.

Digestion: The View from the East

Traditional Chinese medical theory is best understood as both literal and metaphoric. The process of digestion is described as follows: when food is eaten, the stomach receives it and there the food is "rotted and ripened." The spleen separates the "pure" part of the food, which can be thought of as the nutrients it contains. This is sent upward to the lungs, where it is mixed with the energy extracted from the air (think oxygen) and sent to the heart, which distributes the food essence via the blood to nourish the entire body. The spleen is the master organ of digestion in the Chinese medical system, and its job of discerning the nutritive part of the food eaten is vital. The "impure part" of the food is sent downward, toward the small and then the large intestine, which is responsible for removing this waste from the body as the stool.

Not just *what* you eat but also *how* you eat it has a big impact on your digestive function and your energy. The spleen functions best, extracting the most energy from the food you eat, when you eat regularly, slowly, and mindfully and when you chew thoroughly. Science has noted that digestion begins in the brain, when you plan your next meal. Your body starts preparing the appropriate digestive enzymes at this point, known as the *cephalic phase* of digestion (Guyton 1991). The digestive process really gets going in the mouth, as you break up the food by chewing. Most people don't chew enough. There is a Chinese saying: "The stomach has no teeth." You can increase your digestive power and your energy and improve digestive complaints simply with thorough chewing, particularly of fibrous and animal-flesh foods.

EATING FOR THE BEST DIGESTION

Your digestive system is like a soup pot. All food that you take in must be transformed into a 98 degree soup, quite literally. The farther away from soup the food you eat is, the harder your body must work to digest it. Chilled, frozen, and raw foods take more energy to digest. Drinking ice water with meals temporarily shocks the lining of the digestive system, constricting the blood vessels that line its walls and slowing down the soup-making process. The American restaurant custom of serving ice water with meals runs counter to the Chinese medicine view of healthy digestion. If you were making a soup on your stove top and kept adding glassfuls of ice water to the pot, imagine how much longer it would take for your soup to be done!

It's best to drink no more than a small amount of fluid with a meal; save the big glass of water for a between-meal refresher. Room-temperature or warm drinks are best. Many traditional cuisines include the use of fermented beverages at meals, such as wine or beer, or cultured ones, such as beet kvass and lactofermented sodas (see recipes in chapters 2 and 3), which provide digestive enzymes, probiotics, and *lactic acid* (a product of bacterial activity), all of which can enhance digestion. Enjoy beverages in small servings of two to eight ounces with a meal. Eating soup with a meal, or as part of a meal, is a time-honored way to nourish yourself, and research supports its value in increasing satiety: people who eat soup as a first course typically eat fewer calories in total at a meal and later in the same day, and report greater satisfaction with their meals (Rolls et al. 1999; Flood and Rolls 2007).

How strong is your spleen? The spleen is responsible for transforming the food you eat into nutrition for the body, as well transporting these nutrients to where they are needed. The spleen also plays a big role in the fluid metabolism, along with the lungs and the kidneys, and is thought to make the blood of the body. These functions combined connect the strength of the spleen to the strength of our day-to-day energy, and low energy or fatigue is one of the primary symptoms of a weakness in spleen energy. Other symptoms of deficiency of spleen energy include poor appetite, abdominal distension after eating, loose stools, craving sweets, and a tendency to gain weight (Maciocia 1989).

Chinese medicine teaches that sweet foods can strengthen the spleen; however, what is meant by this is naturally sweet foods, such as yams and brown rice, not the foods sweet from refined sugars that make up such a big part of the modern diet. Most grains, vegetables, legumes, dairy, and animal products are classified as having a sweet flavor, and these should form the bulk of the diet, punctuated by foods of other flavors, the effects of which will be described in subsequent chapters. Eating refined sweet foods, particularly refined sugar, in excess can damage the spleen and lead to weakened digestion and symptoms such as fatigue and loose stools.

Eating at regular mealtimes, in a relaxed atmosphere, is a simple way to improve digestion. Chinese medicine advises us to avoid eating too quickly, working or studying while eating, eating in a state of emotional stress, and eating late at night. It is also important not to overwhelm your digestive capacity by overeating. The Japanese repeat a simple reminder before meals: *hara hachi bu,* which means "Eat until you are 80 percent full" (Miller and Sarubin-Fragakis 2008). Your goal is satiety, not fullness. Asian healing traditions teach that emphasizing warm, cooked foods in your diet and choosing simple meals, with a daily serving of soup, will lay the foundation for a strong spleen, good digestion, and abundant energy.

Traditional foods for strengthening the spleen and digestion, available throughout the year, are:

- Whole grains: barley, brown and sweet rice, oats, spelt, millet

- Vegetables: carrots, green beans, leeks, onions, parsnips, pumpkins, turnips, winter squash, yams

- Fruits: berries, cherries, dates, figs (choose dried or frozen fruit when local fresh fruit is not available)

- Spices: caraway, cinnamon, fennel, garlic, ginger, nutmeg

- Beans: black beans, garbanzo beans, peas

- Animal foods: beef, chicken, ham

Digestion: The View from the West

From the viewpoint of Western science, our food provides us with energy, quantified in terms of the calories we consume, with *macronutrients* (fats, carbohydrates, and protein), and with *micronutrients* (vitamins, minerals, and other compounds in small quantities, including chemicals that function as antioxidants). *Calories* are a measure of the heat energy food gives off when burned. Calories are delivered in food in three distinct forms: proteins, which primarily provide body structure but can also be converted to fuel; carbohydrates, which act as our major fuel source; and fats, which serve many purposes in the body, including being used in cell membranes, nerve sheaths, and hormones, as well as energy storage, insulation, and cushioning internal organs. Digestion, therefore, is a mechanical and chemical process that breaks food down into its usable components.

The digestive process begins in the brain, when you anticipate and prepare your next meal. Carbohydrate foods are ingested as starches and sugars, and the digestion of them begins in the mouth, when they are mixed with saliva. When your food reaches the stomach, it is disinfected by the addition of *hydrochloric* (stomach) acid and broken down by muscular churning. Protein digestion begins here with the enzyme *pepsin*, which is activated by the presence of adequate stomach acid. Once converted to a thick, soupy suspension called *chyme*, your food moves to the small intestine, passing by the pancreas, which secretes the majority of enzymes needed for digestion. In the small intestine, carbohydrates, now broken down primarily into glucose, and proteins, in the form of amino acids, are absorbed into the bloodstream, while fats, which require the action of *bile* secreted by the gallbladder to be properly digested, pass first through the lymphatic system and then into the blood.

DIGESTIVE POWER

A few self-help tips for best digestion follow from the above discussion. Adequate chewing of food not only begins the digestion of carbohydrate foods in the mouth but also enhances the entire digestive process. Stomach acid is critical to adequate digestion, and while over-the-counter remedies to suppress it are common, they can cause long-term problems. Research suggests that many people are deficient in stomach acid, especially by middle age (Lipski 2005). Too little stomach acid can cause such common symptoms as bloating and gas after meals, indigestion, diarrhea, and constipation (ibid). Heartburn, caused by stomach acid irritating the esophagus, is often improved by *increasing* stomach acid. Eating fermented foods containing lactic acid (a bacterial by-product), such as fermented vegetables and drinks; consuming salad dressings or sauces made with vinegar or lemon juice; simply taking a little vinegar or lemon juice in water with meals; and eating bitter foods, such as greens, can help augment and/or normalize your production of stomach acid, resulting in better protein digestion and nutrient assimilation.

Eating for Stable Blood Sugar

Maintaining a steady supply of glucose to the brain and optimal amounts in the blood is so important that the body has complex mechanisms to ensure this, including the storage of glucose in the form of *glycogen* in the liver and the ability to create glucose from protein if needed. *Insulin*, secreted by the pancreas, is the hormone that enables your cells to make use of the glucose in your blood for energy. Eating carbohydrate foods that are high in simple sugars, such as sucrose (white sugar and other refined sweeteners), or that are quickly converted to simple sugars by digestive enzymes (white flour and other highly refined grains) creates a large increase in blood glucose, requiring a large release of insulin from the pancreas to help usher the glucose into the cells. *High glycemic* foods are defined as foods that tend to cause a large increase in blood sugar and insulin, promoting energy storage in the form of fat, while *low glycemic* foods cause lower increases and don't tend to promote fat storage.

THE BLOOD SUGAR ROLLER COASTER

The typical North American diet, rich in refined, high glycemic, carbohydrate-filled foods, can create a great strain on the body. Many people eat sweetened and refined foods throughout the day, creating an initial rise in blood sugar, or "sugar high," causing the pancreas to release a rush of insulin, ushering glucose into the cells and creating the familiar "sugar crash," which frequently leads to craving more sugar. If the body releases too much insulin relative to glucose, low blood sugar (*hypoglycemia*) is the result. Hypoglycemia is very uncomfortable, causing such symptoms as fatigue, insomnia, headaches, sweet cravings, nausea, loss of appetite or constant hunger, moodiness, crying spells, irritability, and more (Pitchford 2002). Frequent bouts of hypoglycemia may signal damage to the body's delicate hormonal mechanisms for regulating blood sugar, and, over time, can lead to *insulin resistance* (lack of response by the cells to insulin), weight gain, obesity, and diabetes (Jones 2005).

If your day-to-day energy is less than you'd like, consider whether the culprit is low or unstable blood sugar. In my clinical practice, I have found that when my clients make sure to start the day with breakfast, eat at regular times, transition from refined to whole foods, and choose to eat some fat and protein with every meal and snack, most begin to stabilize their blood sugar and feel much better. These changes also provide sustained, rather than roller-coaster, energy and can help prevent the intense hunger that can lead to sugar cravings and poor food choices. Such changes are often a very important first step for those seeking to improve their overall diets and sense of well-being.

Traditional Food Preparation for Optimal Nutrition

In contrast to modern methods of refining foods, which tend to lower their nutritional value and raise glycemic response, most traditional methods of food processing actually increase nutritional availability and lower glycemic loads (Miller and Sarubin-Fragakis 2008). What are these traditional methods? There are many, but three of the most important are soaking, sprouting, and fermentation. These three techniques all create a kind of predigestion of your food, rendering its nutrients and energy more available to the body.

Soaking and spouting are used around the world in the preparation of mature *seed foods*, which include grains, beans, and nuts and seeds (Steinkraus 1983). Mature seed foods, especially grains, can be difficult to digest, to the benefit of the plant. Look at it from a plant's point of view:

plants package their seeds in forms that will, ideally, be eaten and excreted, but not digested, by animals. An undigested seed, deposited by an animal away from the parent plant (encased in a helpful dose of fertilizer), has a chance to grow and propagate the species. Seed foods have hard, difficult-to-digest coats (the *bran* of grains, which contains most of the fiber) and contain powerful phytochemicals, such as *phytic acid*, that bind up and protect their nutrients. Phytic acid is the storage form of phosphorus in plants, and it easily binds with other minerals, such as calcium, magnesium, zinc, and iron, making them unavailable to whatever or whoever eats them. Soaking and sprouting help to neutralize phytic acid and other inhibitory compounds in seed foods.

Soaking your seed foods before cooking will bring immediate improvements in digestibility and energy. To begin, put whole grains and beans in the conditions they need to sprout—a wet, warm, slightly acidic environment—for a period of time. Soak grains and beans overnight with a splash of lemon juice, vinegar, or *yogurt whey* (an acidic liquid made by draining yogurt) before thoroughly cooking. The same can be done with nuts and seeds, which you may then drain and use in recipes, or dehydrate or roast for storage or use. With a little more time and care, you can sprout grains, beans, and seeds for even more nutritional benefits. You'll find directions for soaking and sprouting in chapter 2.

Fermentation is likely the earliest food preservation technique used by human beings (Mollison 1993), and is used both in combination with soaking and sprouting and on its own. Fermentation is a kind of controlled rotting, where bacteria or yeasts, naturally present in the food, the environment, or introduced by *inoculation* with a culture, are given the conditions they need to grow. *Lactic acid bacteria (LAB)* consume the carbohydrate portion of the food and create organic acids, such as lactic acid, and carbon dioxide. Fermented foods, such as yogurt, sourdough bread, and pickled vegetables, typically have a more moderate effect on blood sugar than their unfermented counterparts. Bacterial fermentation also preserves vitamin C in the original food; synthesizes vitamins B, K, and A and beneficial fatty acids; reduces or eliminates *lactose* (milk sugar, to which many people are intolerant) in dairy foods (Lipski 2005); helps neutralize phytic acid, nitrates, and other potential harmful compounds in foods; and limits the growth of disease-causing bacteria in food. Fermentation also imparts wonderful, complex flavors to foods that cannot be achieved through other forms of food preparation. The art of fermentation is simple to learn, and there are many recipes for fermented foods throughout this book, beginning in chapter 2.

Your Diet, Your Energy

Optimal digestion is the foundation of optimal energy. You are not what you eat, but what you absorb. We'll cover many more ways to strengthen digestion and discuss which foods and preparation techniques are best for each season in the chapters ahead. Before you begin your journey around the wheel of the year, take a few days to assess what your diet is doing for you right now.

Keeping a Food Journal

A food journal is a wonderful way to assess the effects of your diet on your mood and energy levels. While there is no one diet that is suitable for everyone, your body holds the key to understanding which way of eating is best for you. This exercise works best if you follow it during several weekdays and through the weekend, as your eating patterns may change significantly through the week. As you work your way through the chapters and the seasons, return to the food journal again and again as a way to see how your changing diet is affecting you. You can either copy the following chart from the book and carry it with you, or use a small notebook. In the left-hand column, record what you eat and your activities throughout the day. In the right-hand column, indicate your energy levels and moods. You might rate these on a 1 to 10 scale. Also, note any symptoms, such as headaches, bloating, or gas. Looking over a few days of journal entries, observe what patterns emerge. Are you eating at regular times? Skimping on breakfast only to overeat later in the day? Fueling up with caffeine instead of real food? Do certain foods or meals make you feel much worse or much better? Or are you fairly even-keeled throughout the day? There are no right answers here, just the answers you find within yourself. You can return to this exercise in each season or as often as you see fit.

Food Journal   Date

Food/Activity	Time	Energy/Mood
	6:00 a.m.	
	7:00 a.m.	
	8:00 a.m.	
	9:00 a.m.	
	10:00 a.m.	
	11:00 a.m.	
	12:00 p.m.	
	1:00 p.m.	
	2:00 p.m.	
	3:00 p.m.	
	4:00 p.m.	
	5:00 p.m.	
	6:00 p.m.	
	7:00 p.m.	
	8:00 p.m.	
	9:00 p.m.	
	10:00 p.m.	
	11:00 p.m.	

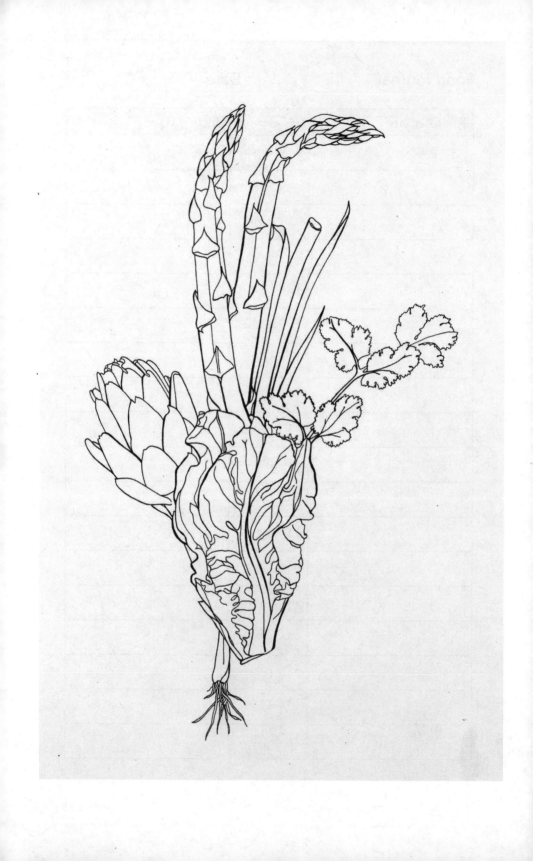

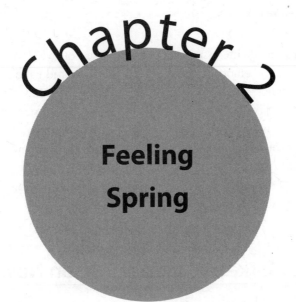

Chapter 2

Feeling Spring

As winter's long nights grow shorter and the wheel of the year spins toward the spring, the earth warms and all life begins to emerge from winter's dormancy. The Chinese lunar calendar calculates the beginning of spring around Chinese New Year, the dates of which vary each year and are usually about six weeks before the equinox. Traditional solar calendars start spring at the equinox, around March 21. The ecological start of spring, of course, will vary with your region and climate. Personally, I celebrate the beginning of spring when the first asparagus of the year appears at the farmers' market, as this signals the beginning of spring produce in my area. If you are in tune with this season, you are refreshed from the internal focus of the winter, and you'll feel energized into new activity. Spring cleaning, for your body as well as your home, is just the thing. If you aren't yet feeling the sense of a spring within, it might be time to adjust your diet to include some of the naturally cleansing foods available now. The farmers' market bursts with foods that help your body clear any internal stagnation you may be experiencing from the reduced activity and overindulgences of winter.

Chinese medicine associates the spring season with the color green, new growth, the emotion of anger, and the liver and gallbladder organs. *The Yellow Emperor's Classic of Medicine* (Ni 1995) reminds us to rise early with the sun, take brisk walks, and breathe in the freshness of the springtime. The coming of spring often brings a sense of restlessness. We long for change, for the new, and nature supports us in seeking renewal at this time of year. The longer days and increased light stimulate your body and mind. The foods of spring, prepared appropriately for the changing climate, provide the nutrients to support this.

At the Market: What's in Season Now

Shopping at the supermarket, where all produce is available year-round, encourages a kind of collective obliviousness to the delights of truly seasonal eating, to the detriment of both our palates and our health. The farther our food travels from harvest to plate, and the more time that elapses, the more of its nutrition is lost. For example, a 2004 study from Purdue University found that fresh spinach lost over 50 percent of its carotenoids and folate after eight days of storage post harvest (Pandrangi and LaBorde 2004). It's time to get reacquainted with the tastes of spring, found in foods such as the shoots and baby greens just beginning to emerge from the warming soil.

In just a generation or two of eating from the supermarket, most of us have lost an intuitive sense of what is in season. In her book *Animal, Vegetable, Miracle*, about a year she and her family spent growing their own food and eating mostly food produced locally, author Barbara Kingsolver offers a wonderful way to help you regain this knowledge: the concept of the *vegetannual*. She asks us to imagine a single plant that bears over the course of the gardening year all the vegetable types that can be harvested and eaten (Kingsolver et al. 2007, 64):

> First, in the early spring, shoots poke up out of the ground. Small leaves appear, then bigger leaves. As the…days grow longer, flower buds will appear, followed by small green fruits. Under midsummer's warm sun, the fruits grow larger, riper, and more colorful. As the days shorten into autumn, these mature into hard-shelled

fruits…. Finally, as the days grow cool, the vegetannual may hoard the sugars its leaves have made, pulling them down into a storage unit of some kind: a tuber, bulb, or root.

In my town the farmers' market is abuzz with excitement the first week of the asparagus harvest, which may begin as early as February and peaks in March and April. Asparagus is a vegetable that epitomizes spring: a tender, green shoot reemerging perennially as the winter fades. Known in Chinese medicine for its cooling and moistening qualities, asparagus is also one of the foods highest in *glutathione*, a powerful antioxidant. Asparagus is traditionally used as an aphrodisiac (in a nod to its phallic appearance, perhaps) and kidney cleanser.

Spring onions, soon followed by green garlic, make their appearance at the market now, and these young shoots replace the mature garlic bulbs and storage onions we have been eating through the winter. Garlic scapes and wild ramps are the very first shoots of these plants, and are a pungent traditional food beginning now to reappear on locally inspired menus. Artichokes, the immature flower buds of the plant, often appear in spring dishes, and it is not a coincidence that they are known to act as a bitter cleansing tonic for the liver. Spring foods are often young, sweet, and tender, as their natural sugars have not yet turned to starch. Indulge in baby carrots, turnips, and beets now and be surprised by their candylike sweetness. And nothing says "spring" like a delicate soup of the season's first English shelling peas in a broth made of their simmered pods.

The animal kingdom is rich in new life and vitality in the spring. Chickens raised on pasture start laying more eggs when the days grow longer, and you may be able to find duck, quail, and chicken eggs of different colors and shapes at the market. As always, when choosing animal products, seek those from sustainably raised animals, ideally from local, small farms. Look for the deep orange-yellow yolks of eggs from chickens raised truly cage-free and able to enjoy a diverse diet, including insects. Independent research conducted by *Mother Earth News* has consistently shown that eggs from chickens raised on pasture are significantly more nutritious than those laid by chickens raised on factory farms. They have "4 to 6 times as much vitamin D…⅓ less cholesterol, ¼ less saturated fat, ⅔ more vitamin A, 2 times more omega-3 fatty acids, 3 times more vitamin E, and 7 times more beta carotene" (Long and Alterman 2007).

The rapidly growing green grass that cows, sheep, and goats graze on at this time of year gives spring milk and cream the distinctive flavors and increased nutrition prized by traditional peoples and chefs around the world. Indulge in some fresh cheese or spring butter from your local farmer and savor the rich taste. Be sure to select dairy products from animals grazing on pasture, not grain. For easiest digestion and maximum nutrition, choose full-fat, *cultured* and/or raw dairy products. Cultured dairy products are those inoculated with a starter culture, usually containing lactic acid bacteria, which proliferate and consume some or all of the milk sugar, or lactose. Thus cultured dairy products are better tolerated by those with lactose intolerance. You'll learn to make crème fraîche at home later in this chapter.

While the safety of raw milk and cheese are controversial in the United States, human beings around the world have been enjoying these nutrient-dense foods for centuries. Raw dairy products are highly nutritious, and have their probiotic and enzyme contents intact, making them easy to digest. The beneficial bacteria in raw dairy can actually help protect against pathogenic bacteria. A recent study found that children who drink raw milk have a significantly lower chance of getting asthma and hay fever than children who don't (Waser et al. 2007).

From the perspective of Chinese medicine, raw and cultured dairy products are more nourishing and less likely to weaken the spleen than their pasteurized counterparts. Like many raw foods, raw milk does pose a small risk of infection, typically from *listeria* bacteria. However, in a joint report by the FDA, USDA, and CDC in 2003, the three government agencies estimated, on a per-serving basis, that deli meats and hot dogs were nearly ten times more dangerous than raw milk (FDA/USDA 2003). While I advise my clients and family members to choose raw milk and dairy products where they are available, I caution against it for people with depressed immunity, such as pregnant women, or those with immature immune systems, such as very young children.

Spring Cooking

Spring cooking styles should shift from the warming techniques of winter, employing shorter cooking times, lower temperatures, and less oil. Think sauté, steam, blanch, and simmer instead of stew, fry, roast, or bake. Use oils more as condiments than for cooking. The warming weather makes raw foods and fresh salads seem newly appealing. As the weather warms, consider gradually increasing the percentage of raw food in your diet. Spring is the time for planting your annual vegetable garden or at least starting a batch of sprouts in a mason jar next to your kitchen sink. Sprouting is a wonderful way to grow your own fresh, nutrient-rich food at home, and sprouted foods are especially energizing in springtime. Later in this chapter are techniques and recipes for growing your own sprouts.

Now is also a good time to increase the fermented foods in your diet. Sauerkraut, kimchi, and other pickles; dairy ferments such as yogurt and kefir, another type of cultured milk; *umeboshi* plum vinegar (a raw vinegar with a salty/sour taste); and fermented drinks, including kombucha and beet kvass, are like *super-raw foods*, providing the enzymatic benefits of raw food plus the support of beneficial bacteria. Make a practice of eating a little fermented food each day or with each meal; this will renew your intestinal flora *and* your energy. Find fermented foods such as these in a natural foods market, or follow the recipes in this chapter to learn to make simple fermented foods at home.

Delicious, Cleansing Greens

We all know greens are good for you. Many greens taste their best now, as winter turns into spring, with the sturdy cooking greens showing a delightful sweetness even as the spicy, sour, and bitter young greens of the season are pushing out of the ground to nudge them aside. Traditional peoples set out to gather the new leaves of spring, such as dandelion greens and nettles, in a ritual of taking spring tonics that we moderns would do well to continue. Many of the young spring greens are crisp and tender, and may have a bitter, sour, or spicy bite: think arugula, sorrel, watercress, baby bok choy, mâche, and endive. Greens were likely one of the most reliable foods of humans during our evolution, as they can be grown and foraged in most climates much of the year. Our systems run well when we munch on a steady supply of greens. Greens' natural bitterness moves energy in the body and stimulates the gallbladder to release bile, aiding in fat and protein digestion, and their high vitamin, mineral, and fiber content comes with beneficial fatty acids and very few calories.

All greens are healthy, but not all are equally nutritious. To sort out their different nutritional and cooking qualities, it helps to think of them in families. The basic groups of greens to be aware of include the cabbage (*Brassica*) family; the spinach/chard (*Amaranthaceae*) family; the lettuces; the leafy green herbs such as basil, parsley and cilantro; and the wild "weeds" like dandelion leaf, sorrel, and purslane.

The cabbage family greens are perhaps the best known of all greens. This large family includes not only the familiar cabbages, kale, broccoli, collard greens, watercress, and kohlrabi, but also radishes, turnips and their greens, mustard greens, and that gourmet favorite, arugula. Greens in this family generally provide plenty of vitamin C, potassium, calcium, vitamin B6, biotin, magnesium, and manganese (Murray et al. 2005). They are most famous for their high phytochemical content, including *sulfuraphanes*, particularly noted for their cancer-protective effects. On the side of caution, however, it has been observed in animal studies that this family of vegetables can exert thyroid-suppressing effects (Masterjohn 2007). These *goitrogenic* compounds are reduced by cooking, particularly boiling. Traditional diets that are high in cabbage-family vegetables, such as Japanese diets, usually incorporate iodine-containing foods such as fish, seafood, and sea vegetables, which can help protect the thyroid.

Another fantastic feature of the cabbage family is that these vegetables are so amenable to fermentation, especially the cabbages and other leafy greens. The *probiotics*, or health-enhancing bacteria, that live on the greens will happily proliferate when you give them the right conditions, as when you make sauerkraut, kimchi, or *curtido*, increasing the digestibility of your greens, enhancing their flavor, and strengthening your immune system. See the recipes later in this chapter.

Spinach, chard, and beet greens are all from the same family, known botanically as *Amaranthaceae*, or the amaranth family. These greens share the qualities of tender mouthfeel and quick cooking. Don't throw away the greens that may be attached to your beets! These types of greens are high in vitamin K, chlorophyll, carotenes, vitamin C, and folic acid, and have some manganese, magnesium, iron, and vitamin B2. However, they are also high in oxalic acid, which binds to the iron and calcium in the greens and other foods eaten at the same meal so that much less of these important minerals are usable by the body (Murray et al. 2005). One study found a reduction of available calcium in such greens of 15 to 95 percent (Radek and Savage 2008). If you've ever felt a gritty sensation on your teeth after eating raw spinach, you've noticed this effect. Cooking or eating spinach and related greens with other foods high in calcium, such as dairy foods, can inactivate the oxalates. Another strategy is to use a variety of greens in your cooking to minimize the downside of any one family of greens. For example, in recipes calling for spinach, try a mix of spinach and arugula for more balanced nutrition and complex flavor.

Lettuce, queen of salad greens, is classified into four categories: iceberg, or crisp head, lettuce, the pale, round solid heads that still comprise many an American salad; romaine, with its deep-green, long leaves and stronger flavor and texture; butterhead, featuring large, tender leaves forming a loose head (think Boston and Bibb lettuce); and leaf, which has broad and curly leaves arranged in a loose, conic head (red leaf, green leaf). In general, as with most leafy greens, the darker and stronger tasting the lettuce, the greater its nutrient content.

All lettuce provides chlorophyll and vitamin K. Romaine is the most nutrient rich of the lettuces, with ten to one hundred times the vitamins and phytonutrients of iceberg. Romaine lettuce is an excellent source of vitamin A, C, B1, and B2; folic acid; manganese; and chromium. Lettuce is primarily water, and commercial lettuce is notorious for high pesticide residues, so go for organic whenever you can. Of course, there are many other tender greens outside of the lettuce family that can be used in salads, like arugula, mizuna, frisée, and watercress. Most of these are in the cabbage family and offer superb nutrition as well as taste.

Leafy green culinary herbs such as parsley, cilantro, mint, and basil are available year-round in many areas but reach their peak now through summer. What nutritional powerhouses they are! Culinary herbs and spices are where food and medicine really come together. Parsley is a great example. The plant is a member of the *Umbelliferae* family, along with the culinary aromatic superstars carrots, celery, and fennel and close cousin cilantro. Parsley is a very good source of vitamins A and C, folic acid, and minerals such as iron, magnesium, calcium, potassium, and zinc. The volatile oils in parsley, such as myristicin, are cancer-protective, while the many *flavonoids* (plant compounds that impart vivid pigments) it contains, especially luteolin, are powerful antioxidants that help prevent oxygen-related damage to your cells (Mateljan 2001).

Wild weeds, such as dandelion leaves, seem to pop up everywhere in spring. Your garden, or a neighbor's, can likely supply you with some. (Who says there's no free lunch?) Dandelion leaf is known to herbalists as a liver tonic, a rich source of vitamins and minerals, and it has a daringly bitter taste. Your garden or a nearby wild place may also be a great place to pick some nutritious "weeds" like chickweed, miner's lettuce, sorrel, nettles, or purslane, which is very high in anti-inflammatory omega-3 fatty acids. Nasturtium leaves are a spicy, abundant "weed" in my garden, and the leaves and flowers pepper many of my lunchtime salads, while I pickle the seedpods in brine to make "poor man's capers." Wild greens are generally higher in nutrient content than their domesticated counterparts (Miller and Sarubin-Fragakis 2008), but be sure to forage only from clean places far from busy roads, as plants pick up chemicals from their environments.

Twelve Ways to Get More Greens into Your Life

1. Add a side of sturdy cooked greens or a handful of leafy salad to your breakfast. Make a habit of always making a double batch of cooked greens and reserving half for future meals.

2. Stir chopped parsley or cilantro into soups and stews, and use them to garnish salads or almost any dish.

3. Any cooking greens can enhance a frittata, a dish that works for breakfast, lunch, or dinner and makes great leftovers! Or simply scramble greens and eggs for a quick meal.

4. Use spinach, arugula, or watercress on your next sandwich to get a nutrient boost beyond what lettuce gives.

5. Make a batch of green soup, eat it with any meal, and freeze some for another day; recipes start later in this chapter.

6. Make green pesto; go beyond basil by adding spinach, arugula, kale, or other greens to your next batch, and use it as a garnish for soup, scrambled eggs, or roasted veggies. See the recipes later in this chapter. Every culinary tradition seems to have condiments based on fresh, green herbs, such as the Italian *salsa verde,* Latin *chimichurri,* and fresh Indian chutneys; seek them out to add to your repertoire.

7. Here's a lunch staple: a large green salad with leftover cooked veggies and meat, beans, or cheese for protein power can be made quickly at home and can travel with you to work or school. Dress it at the last minute with your homemade salad dressing (recipes come later in this chapter).

8. Learn to identify wild edible greens and enjoy a handful on your next hike.

9. Refresh leftover soups or beans with a big handful of finely chopped kale, collards, or other cooking greens. Simmer until tender, garnish with chopped parsley, and add a spoonful of pesto for triple-green power.

10. Microgreens (young greens harvested when they are less than an inch high) are potent in flavor and nutrition, make an elegant garnish, and are becoming more available in markets. Or go one step beyond sprouting and learn to grow your own.

11. Drink your greens. Add a handful of any type of greens to your next smoothie. Freshly juice greens with other produce, or brew a tea of nettles, mint, or raspberry leaf.

12. Make a practice of adding leafy greens to every meal, especially in the spring.

Spring Renewal: How the Health of Your Liver Affects Your Energy

The ancient wisdom of Chinese medicine teaches us to attend to the health of the liver and its companion organ, the gallbladder, in the spring. The understanding of the liver in Chinese medicine is similar to, but broader than, the view of the liver in Western physiology. According to Chinese medicine, the liver is responsible for keeping energy and emotions moving in the body, for storing and purifying the blood, for the health of the eyes, and for the strength and suppleness of the tendons and nails (Pitchford 2002).

Chinese medical thinking associates the liver with the emotion of anger, and it is considered the master organ of all the emotions. The liver's main job in this regard is maintaining emotional flow. The major emotions described in the Chinese medicine literature are anger, sadness, fear, joy, and worry. They are all healthy and may be appropriate responses to various situations in life, but when we get stuck in one emotional state, disharmony, followed by disease, may strike. The key to emotional health, therefore, is to let the emotional life flow. The most common way the liver gets out of balance is through stagnation, when its ability to keep the flow going becomes compromised. The overloaded liver shows a pattern called liver qi stagnation in Chinese medicine, an extremely common syndrome among modern people. Symptoms of liver qi stagnation include a feeling of bloating or discomfort in the torso, moodiness, edginess, frustration, sadness or depression, PMS, and irregular menstruation (Maciocia 1989).

The best way to adjust your diet to relieve liver qi stagnation is to eat smaller amounts of congestive foods, including animal foods, nuts, and nut butter, and to eat less food altogether. People with liver qi stagnation often crave caffeine, alcohol, or hot, spicy food, which gives a temporary feeling of relief but ultimately adds to the problem. Increasing the amount of raw and super-raw fermented foods in your diet can help get energy moving and make you feel less stuck and more vital. Specific seasonal foods that will get liver energy moving include pungent foods and aromatic herbs, such as the following:

- Herbs and spices: anise, basil, bay, cardamom, cayenne and white pepper (in small quantities), cinnamon, cloves, cilantro, curry, fennel, garlic, ginger, horseradish, mint, mustard, nutmeg, oregano, parsley, vanilla

- Beans: navy, baby lima, cannellini, and other white beans

- Vegetables: collard greens, green garlic, kohlrabi, leeks, onions, radishes of all types, turnips and their greens, watercress

- Fruits: grapefruit, lemon, lime, kumquat, early plums, tangerine

The Liver in Western Medicine

Western physiology views your liver as both your body's chemical factory and a major recycling center. Each day thousands of chemical reactions go on in this organ as it processes nutrients from food, creates and breaks down hormones and enzymes, and handles chemicals from your diet and environment. While *detoxification* activities happen throughout your body, the majority occur in your liver. Detoxification is what your body does to get rid of unwanted chemicals, be they leftovers of your own metabolism, stress hormones, products of your intestinal bacteria, or substances you eat, breathe, or rub into your skin or hair. There are two phases in your body's detoxification process. The first, phase I, involves various reactions, usually involving liver enzymes, such as those in the cytochrome P450 family, which render foreign molecules easier to remove from the body. In phase II, these new molecules (some of which may be more toxic than the original compounds) are removed from the body via urine and stool. Detoxification reactions require many nutrients, such as B vitamins, glutathione, flavonoids, and phospholipids in phase I, and amino acids including glutamine, taurine, glycine, and methionine in phase II (Jones 2005)—nutrients that are scarce in refined foods but abundant in many whole foods, particularly, in the case of the amino acids, in pasture-raised eggs and animal foods.

Spring Cleaning for Your Home and Body

Integrative physician Sidney Baker, in his 2003 book *Detoxification and Healing*, estimates that over 80 percent of our daily energy is used by the body for detoxification activities. If you can reduce your body's need for detoxification, you can liberate more energy for other purposes. The foods you choose can either add to your body's workload or support it in its efforts to keep things running smoothly. Foods that require more energy for your body to process include rancid or hydrogenated fats; burned or charbroiled foods; foods that contain artificial colors, flavors, or preservatives; and highly refined foods, including white sugar and white flour. Eating too many of these foods, being exposed to more chemicals than the body can handle, or simply living with too much stress can create a backlog that can result in uncomfortable symptoms.

Government and independent testing has shown that virtually *all* of us carry synthetic chemicals in our bodies (Thornton et al. 2002). The available scientific literature documents the presence of over two hundred chemical compounds in the bodies of the general public—people with no special history of chemical exposure. When the body is unable to detoxify foreign compounds due to their nature or to overloaded detoxification systems, they are simply stored in the tissues, where they accumulate. The sum total of chemicals each of us carries is termed our *body burden*. While it is impossible to avoid exposure to many of these potentially toxic compounds, you *can* choose cleaner sources of food and select nontoxic products for your body, home, and garden to greatly reduce your daily chemical load. Make it a goal in this year's spring cleaning to switch to clean and green household products and cosmetics, and clear out the chemicals under the sink or in the garage, taking anything hazardous to your community's hazardous disposal site.

The following chart will assist you in reducing the chemical load of your diet:

Instead of...	Choose...
• Factory-farmed animal foods	• Pastured and/or organic animal foods
• Factory-farmed fish and seafood	• Sustainably harvested wild or sustainably farmed fish and seafood
• Low-fat and nonfat homogenized, pasteurized dairy products	• Full-fat, nonhomogenized or cream-top, organic, and raw or cultured dairy products
• Margarine, partially hydrogenated vegetable oils, and most commercial vegetable oils	• Expeller-pressed olive, sesame, coconut, or palm kernel oil; organic butter, ghee, or pastured lard
• Supermarket produce	• Organic and/or local produce
• White flour, bread, pasta, and rice	• Whole grain flour, bread, pasta, and rice, preferably prepared using soaking or fermenting techniques where applicable
• White sugar, sucrose, high-fructose corn syrup, and dextrose	• Unrefined cane sugar, raw honey, or maple syrup
• Iodized, refined salt	• Unrefined sea salt
• Soy milk, tofu, and soy protein isolates	• Fermented traditional soy products such as tempeh, miso, and tamari
• Bottled water	• Filtered tap water
• Artificial food colorings and flavorings, MSG, aspartame, saccharin, and Splenda	• Nonirradiated herbs and spices, bone broths, tamari, fish sauce, unrefined sweeteners, stevia
• Synthetic vitamins and supplements	• Food-based vitamins and supplements if necessary

Lightening Your Toxic Load

There are many dietary strategies that can help reduce your absorption of toxins and assist your body in removing them. Sufficient intake of fats, protein, carbohydrates, and vitamins and minerals protects us from absorbing environmental toxins and assists the immune system in recognizing and removing them from our bodies (Jones 2005). When the body is depleted of minerals, for example, toxic metals are more likely to be taken up and incorporated into cells. Of course, many people are deficient in vitamins and minerals. Industrial agriculture depletes the soils and has resulted in lower nutritional value of most crops since the 1930s (Davis 2009). Refined sugar, flour, and oils; caffeine, nicotine, alcohol, and drugs; and food additives of all types act to deplete the body's vitamin and mineral stores and overburden our natural detoxification systems. It makes sense to choose to avoid substances like these, which are known nutrient depleters.

Many raw and lightly cooked foods, including avocado, walnuts, grapefruits, spinach, and tomatoes are whole food sources of glutathione (Murray et al. 2005) used by the body to convert fat-soluble toxins into water-soluble compounds for excretion. Glutathione requires sufficient vitamin B6, riboflavin, and selenium to be effective. Another of the major detoxification systems in phase II requires sulfur (abundant in beans, eggs, cabbage family vegetables, and meat). *Ellagic acid*, an antioxidant that helps your body detoxify many airborne pollutants, is destroyed by heat. It is abundant in raspberries and blackberries, and is also found in other berries, most fruits, and nuts, such as walnuts and pecans. Fiber is found in most whole foods and helps to eliminate heavy metals as well, although excess fiber, as from fiber supplements, can block mineral absorption.

CLEANSING TRADITIONS

Many traditional diets include periodic cleanses or modified fasts that can reduce the toxic load and support the body in renewing itself. In her book *The Jungle Effect* (Miller and Sarubin-Fragakis 2008), Daphne Miller describes how people practicing Greek Orthodox holiday fasts on Crete had both lower body mass and lower LDL cholesterol, effects that persisted throughout the year. A 2002 study showed that a traditional Ayurvedic cleanse, based on the use of ghee, was even able to reduce the body burden of the hard-to-remove chemicals polychlorinated biphenyls, or PCBs (Herron and Fagan 2002).

The body requires an array of nutrients for detoxification, so simplifying your diet for a period of time is safer and more effective than more extreme programs, like water fasting or the master cleanse, a regimen consisting of water mixed with maple syrup, lemon juice, and cayenne pepper. Chinese medicine has traditionally warned against complete or water fasting. *The Yellow Emperor's Classic of Medicine* (Maciocia 1989, 51) states: "After a half day of fasting, the qi weakens, and after a full day of fasting, it is very low." When you avoid food entirely for too long, your body must draw on deep nutrient reserves, which can be damaging.

A very simple one-day cleanse can be done by eating raw fruit for breakfast, a large salad for lunch, and a simple broth-based soup for dinner. Try a bowl of Spring Green Soup (later in this chapter) for breakfast. A longer cleanse of several days to several weeks can effectively relieve symptoms such as those listed in the box, get stuck energy moving, and bring you to a more vibrant state of health and attunement with the energy of spring.

A *simple spring cleanse* can clear many major and minor symptoms and bring you a sense of renewed energy. You can use the same protocol at other times of the year, but substitute the appropriate seasonal produce. This process becomes even more powerful when you work with an herbalist or naturopath to include foods and herbs specific for your condition. Also, if you suspect food sensitivities or allergies, you can test them effectively when you add foods back in after the cleansing process. A week or two before cleansing, begin your preparations. First, reduce your caffeine intake gradually. If you drink coffee, start mixing water-processed decaf with regular coffee until you are down to pure decaf. The week before you cleanse, make or purchase fermented foods such as kombucha, sauerkraut, kimchi, *curtido*, or other pickled veggies, and beet kvass (see recipes starting later in this chapter). Clean out your cupboards of processed, packaged, and other unhealthy foods. Finally, have a last fling with foods not on the program, if you feel the need.

Refrain from: alcohol, caffeine, grains (except brown or wild rice and quinoa), nuts and seeds (except flax meal), dairy except for organic ghee, all packaged and refined foods, and refined sugar.

Self-Quiz: Would You Benefit from Cleansing?

How many of the following have you experienced in the last two months?

Allergies

Skin rashes or breakouts

Tight neck and shoulders

Headaches

Constipation, loose stools, or both

Difficulty falling or staying asleep

PMS

Menstrual cramps

Restlessness, irritability, or anger

Mood swings

Frequent infections or colds

Poor memory or mental fogginess

If you have had more than two or three of these symptoms regularly, chances are you would benefit from following a simple food-based cleanse like the following one. If you have had five or more of them consistently, please consult with a health care provider before beginning such a program.

Choose:

- Vegetables. Eat all types, as much as you wish. Raw vegetables are more cleansing; cooked ones are more strengthening. People who are robust and those cleansing in warmer climates can choose more raw foods (50 percent or more); those who are tired or deficient and those cleansing in cool weather should choose more cooked foods (75 percent or more).

- Cleansing vegetables. Eat at least two of the following per day: avocados, artichokes, asparagus, beets, broccoli, Brussels sprouts, burdock, cabbage, carrots, cauliflower, celery, chives, cucumbers, eggplant, garlic, jicama, kohlrabi, leeks, mushrooms, onions, peppers, rutabaga, radishes (especially daikon and Spanish black radish), sea vegetables, and turnips.

- Leafy greens. Eat all types, such as arugula, beet, daikon, and turnip greens; dandelion greens; kale and collard greens; mustard greens; Swiss chard; spinach; lettuce of all types; and edible flowers.

- Fruit. Choose any fresh or frozen fruit, with an emphasis on seasonal fruits from your area. Try to eat at least twice as many vegetables as fruits. No dried or canned fruit.

- Fats and oils. Choose only expeller-pressed organic olive oil, unrefined coconut oil or ghee, or pastured lard for cooking, and organic expeller-pressed flax oil and olive oil for dressing salads.

- Beans. Eat one to three servings of organic lentils, mung beans, chickpeas, or other beans daily. Soak all beans overnight before cooking. Avoid unfermented soy (tofu or soy milk), but tempeh and *shoyu* or tamari are okay.

- Grains (optional). Eat one to three servings of organic brown rice, wild rice, or quinoa daily, and prepare them by soaking overnight before cooking.

- Animal foods. Choose from organic or pastured poultry, beef, lamb, or goat and wild-caught, low-mercury seafood only, up to four 2- to 3-ounce servings per day. Eat one to three organic or pastured eggs daily. Prepare animal products by boiling, baking, roasting, or poaching. No cured, smoked, or preserved meats, but canned salmon and sardines are okay if your budget is tight.

- Seasonings. Choose natural wheat-free tamari or shoyu, chickpea miso (available at natural foods groceries), raw apple cider vinegar or other raw vinegars, fresh lemon juice, Celtic sea salt or other unprocessed salt, fresh or dried organic herbs and spices, raw honey, and nutritional yeast.

- Fermented foods. Eat raw sauerkraut or lactofermented pickles, ideally with each meal.

- Beverages. Aim for half your body weight in ounces of water a day (average is eight to ten glasses), more if you exercise vigorously. Choose filtered water, herbal teas, kombucha, and beet kvass; freshly pressed vegetable juices; or freshly pressed fruit juices diluted with water.

Continue cleansing for three days to four weeks. You may want to start with a short cleanse and work up to longer ones. You may continue regular, moderate exercise during this time, or add daily brisk walks if you have been sedentary. Massage, acupuncture, saunas, and dry skin brushing are useful adjuncts to a cleansing diet (Ohlgren and Tomasulo 2006). While many people experience increasing energy and vitality while cleansing, it is also common to have flulike symptoms, including nausea, headaches, tiredness, aches and pains, and the return of old symptoms of various types, all of which usually pass within a day or two. When you return to normal eating, do so gradually. It is wise to reintroduce foods one group at a time, and you can check for reactions to any food groups to which you think you might be sensitive, such as wheat or dairy. Eat from each new food group a few times and wait a day or two to check for reactions before adding the next.

Spring Recipes

In this section you'll find recipes for staple foods and cooking techniques that will be used many times in the recipes that follow in later chapters, such as basic fermentation, culturing, sprouting, and making ghee. You'll also be tempted to celebrate the fresh flavors of spring with dishes that feature ingredients that are at their best at this time of year, and that will help cleanse and reinvigorate your body after a long winter.

The recipes draw on diverse culinary traditions, yet teach techniques found around the world. Many of these methods of food preparation have been abandoned in the last fifty years as people have embraced the use of store-bought foods and culinary shortcuts. While the recipes in this book can be made with a minimum of kitchen equipment, you'll find that having the following items will make your time in the kitchen a lot more enjoyable.

- Sharp knife. A good-quality carbon-steel blade will serve you well for nearly a lifetime. Keep it sharp by getting yourself a sharpening stone and learning to use it, and your chopping tasks will be a pleasure.

- Cast-iron skillet. The original nontoxic, nonstick pot, cast iron cooks with even, steady heat, adds iron to your food, and cleans up in a breeze.

- Large soup/stockpot. Essential for making convenient stocks and broths and large batches of soup to serve and freeze.

- Slow cooker. Most households already have one. Put yours to work making stocks and broths while you sleep, or cooking dinner while you are at work. I use mine a few times a week for pots of beans, bone broths, and braised meats.

- Handheld immersion blender. This allows soup, the staff of life, to be made in a jiffy, while saving you chopping and cleanup time. Purée foods right in the pot in which you cooked them.

- Microplane grater/zester. No, it's not cheap, but you'll never zest citrus or grate hard cheeses with more pleasure and ease.

- Food processor. This sure makes life easier sometimes, but it is by no means mandatory. I use my handheld immersion blender a lot more often.

- Mason jars (1- and 2-quart sizes). Mason jars are the fermenter's friends; they're also great nonplastic storage for leftovers and staples.

You might notice that all of the recipes in this book are gluten-free. While this is not a book about gluten-free diets, gluten allergy and intolerance are health issues for many people today. For many others, refined flour- and wheat-based foods comprise the bulk of calorie intake and are relatively low in nutrition. Most people will experience health benefits from shifting their diets toward traditional nutrient-dense foods such as the animal foods; seasonal produce; and beans, nuts, and seeds featured in the following recipes.

Spring Shopping List

Animal Products: pastured chicken, duck, lamb, eggs, full-fat raw or pastured milk and cheese, goat's milk and cheese, cultured dairy products, including butter, yogurt, and kefir

Grains: wheat, rye, brown basmati, and long-grain brown rice

Vegetables: artichokes, arugula, asparagus, avocados, baby bok choy, baby greens of lettuces and other vegetables, beets, cardoons, carrots, English peas, fava beans, fennel, green garlic, green onions, leeks, nettles, nopales (cactus paddles), spring onions, pea shoots, radishes, rhubarb, snap peas, snow peas, sorrel, sprouts, turnips, watercress

Fruits: cherries, grapefruit, kumquats, lemons, mandarins, strawberries

Herbs, Spices, and Condiments: cilantro, mint, parsley, and other fresh herbs; apple cider vinegar and/or umeboshi plum vinegar; raw sauerkraut, kimchi, and other fermented vegetables

Sauerkraut

This most basic of vegetable ferments can be varied with many seasonal additions. You can ferment it for three days, three weeks, or three months, depending on your patience and taste.

Makes 1 quart

1 head cabbage

2 teaspoons fine sea salt

1 teaspoon caraway, fennel, or mustard seeds, fresh or dry dill, or juniper berries

With a knife or box grater, shred the cabbage as finely as you can and place it in a large bowl. Sprinkle the salt over the cabbage and massage it in, squeezing until the cabbage begins to exude some juice and the color darkens a bit. Once it is thoroughly wet, add the spices and mix thoroughly. Stuff the cabbage into a wide-mouthed 1-quart mason jar, pressing down with your hands so that the cabbage juice rises above the level of the shredded cabbage. Use a smaller jar or bottle that will fit inside the mouth of the jar to keep the cabbage weighted down and covered by its juice as it ferments. Place the jar on a saucer to catch any drips, and cover the whole thing with a kitchen towel secured with a rubber band.

Allow to ferment at room temperature for 3 days or more. Check the sauerkraut each day to be sure the cabbage is submerged and to taste it to see if it has achieved a flavor you like. When you feel it is ready, seal the lid and refrigerate to slow further fermentation. Eat 1 teaspoon or more with every meal.

Yogurt Whey and Yogurt Cream Cheese

Draining yogurt yields two very useful products. Use the cheese as you would a thick yogurt or cream cheese, or blend with herbs to make a savory dip. Use the whey in making Beet Kvass (on the next page), Rosemary Lemonade (chapter 3), or Hibiscus and Rose Hip Soda (chapter 3); add a teaspoon of whey to soaking grains or beans to improve their digestibility; or drink it straight as a digestive tonic.

Makes about 1½ cups of yogurt whey and 2½ cups of yogurt cream cheese

1 quart whole-milk organic yogurt

Place a colander over a large bowl. Line it with a tea towel or very fine cheesecloth, and pour in the yogurt. Cover and let drain at room temperature 8 to 24 hours. When it has achieved a consistency you like, pour the whey into a small jar and scrape the yogurt cheese off the towel into a container of your choice. The cream cheese will keep in the refrigerator for a few weeks, the whey for up to 6 weeks.

Beet Kvass

This drink is valuable for its medicinal qualities and as a digestive aid. Beets are just loaded with nutrients. One four-ounce glass, morning and night, is an excellent blood tonic, cleanses the liver, and is a good treatment for kidney stones and other ailments. Beet kvass may also be used in place of vinegar in salad dressings and as an addition to soups. This recipe is adapted from Sally Fallon's version, in her book *Nourishing Traditions* (2000). Chop the beets for kvass; don't grate them. When grated, beets exude too much juice, resulting in a too-rapid fermentation that favors the production of alcohol over lactic acid.

Makes 2 quarts

3 medium or 2 large organic beets, chopped up coarsely

¼ cup Yogurt Whey (see previous page)

1½ teaspoons sea salt

Filtered water

Place the beets, whey, and salt in a 2-quart glass container. Add filtered water to fill the container. Stir well and cover securely. Keep at room temperature for 2 days before transferring to the refrigerator, where it will keep for up to 2 months.

When most of the liquid has been drunk, you may fill up the container with water and keep it at room temperature another 2 days. The resulting brew will be slightly less strong than the first. After the second brew, discard the beets and start again. You may, however, reserve some of the liquid and use this as your inoculant instead of the whey.

Crème Fraîche

This easily made cultured cream has a wonderful mild flavor and will add probiotics, beneficial fats, and enzymes to any dish calling for cream, milk, yogurt, or sour cream. You can use any of several types of cultured dairy as an inoculant including crème fraîche itself. It can also be whipped and used as a dessert topping, or drained as in making yogurt cheese (earlier in this chapter) to make your own mascarpone. Be sure to use cream from cows that have been fed on pasture, and enjoy it in the spring for the biggest concentration of fat-soluble vitamins, such as A and D.

Makes about 1½ cups

1 tablespoon organic buttermilk, crème fraîche, or plain yogurt

1½ cups organic heavy (whipping) cream

Place the buttermilk in a pint jar and add the cream. Gently stir them together, cap, and allow to ferment in a warm place (such as on top of the refrigerator) for 1 to 2 days, until the crème fraîche begins to firm. Store it in the refrigerator and consume within 2 weeks.

Ghee

Ghee is easily made at home. Spring is the best time to stock up because of the extra nutrients in the butter produced by cows grazing on fresh green grass. It is stable up to moderately high temperatures, imparts wonderful flavor to foods, will keep for months without refrigeration, and is thought to be both nourishing and digestion-enhancing in Ayurveda, the traditional healing system of India.

Makes about 2 cups

1 pound organic, unsalted butter, preferably from cows raised on pasture

Put the butter in a pan with a heavy bottom, such as a cast-iron skillet. Turn the heat to medium and allow the butter to melt. When you see bubbles begin to rise to the top, turn the heat down to medium-low and allow the butter to cook, uncovered. You'll see whitish curds form at the bottom of the pot. After about 10 minutes, you'll notice a lovely aroma, like popcorn, being released from the ghee, which will begin to turn clear except for the whitish curds that are forming. Watch it carefully, and stir to ensure that it does not burn. If the curds begin to brown, reduce the heat or remove the pan from the heat altogether, as this is a sign that it is about to burn.

When the ghee is clear, after 15 to 20 minutes total, remove it from the heat. Let it cool until just warm, about 5 minutes, and then strain the ghee into a jar through a fine-mesh strainer lined with several layers of cheesecloth or a tea towel. You can use the strained-out milk solids as a vegetable topping, or to impart a buttery flavor to bread or pancake batter. Store the ghee at room temperature; it will keep indefinitely.

Herb Pesto

Pesto is a versatile condiment and a great way to get the nutritional benefits of greens along with a dose of probiotics and beneficial fats. Either the traditional Parmesan or white miso (available at natural food stores and Asian markets) adds a deep, savory flavor as well as digestive enzymes. You don't need to wait for basil season to enjoy pesto, as it can be made with a variety of herbs. Try sage, arugula, oregano, or marjoram. Pesto is also a great way to use the stems of parsley and cilantro when you have used the leaves for other dishes. Serve it atop Spring Green Soup, a dish of beans, scrambled eggs, or roasted vegetables, or dilute it with lemon juice and use it as a salad dressing.

Makes 1½ cups

½ cup raw, unsalted walnuts, almonds, or other nuts
1 bunch parsley, coarsely chopped (stems okay)
1 bunch basil or cilantro (stems okay)
1 clove garlic or 2 tablespoons coarsely chopped green garlic
¼ cup extra-virgin olive oil
Juice of 1 or 2 lemons
2 tablespoons freshly grated Parmesan cheese or 2 tablespoons white or chickpea miso

Sea salt

Soak the nuts overnight in water to cover.

The next morning, drain the nuts, discarding the soaking water. Place them in your food processor or blender and process into a fine paste. Add the parsley, cilantro, and garlic and process until finely ground. Add the olive oil and process until incorporated, and then add lemon juice and more salt if needed to get a flavor you like. Store the pesto in an airtight container in the fridge for up to 10 days, or freeze for several months.

Spring Green Soup

This soup evokes spring in color and taste, and eating it for breakfast, lunch, or dinner can make you feel a sense of springtime within. I like to eat it with a big spoonful of sauerkraut, green pesto, or crème fraîche and a slice of sourdough rye bread and butter for a quick and easy spring meal. Leftovers freeze well. Add a big handful of chopped greens to freshen it when you reheat it. Most varieties of leafy greens, such as spinach, kale, turnip and mustard greens; arugula; nettles; or a combination of these, work well in this soup. You'll want to adjust your cooking time, depending on how thick or fibrous the greens you choose.

Serves 4 to 6

2 tablespoons ghee, lard, coconut oil, or olive oil

1 bunch spring or green onions, white and green parts, coarsely chopped

½ cup fennel or celery, coarsely chopped

1 quart Bone Broth (page 138), Poultry Stock (page 115), Savory Vegetable Broth (page 139), or water

2 small potatoes or turnips, diced into ½-inch cubes

1 bunch leafy greens, such as spinach or arugula, coarsely chopped (about 2 cups)

1 teaspoon fresh or dried dill

2 tablespoons chickpea miso or white miso

Juice of 1 lemon

Heat the ghee or other fat in a medium soup pot over moderate heat. When the fat just begins to liquefy, add the onions and sauté until their edges begin to turn golden, 2 to 3 minutes. Add the fennel or celery and sauté a few minutes more. Add the stock or water and turnips, turn the heat to high, and bring the soup to a boil. Cover the pot and reduce the heat to simmer for 15 minutes. Add the greens and continue to simmer until all the vegetables are tender, for 5 to 15 minutes more depending on the varieties of greens you choose. Turn off the heat and stir in the dill and the miso. Purée the soup with an immersion blender, or allow it to cool and purée in batches in a blender or food processor. Stir in the lemon juice and taste the soup. You're looking for a balance of bitter, tart, salty, and aromatic flavors. Adjust the seasonings as needed.

Basic Sprouting Method

Many whole, raw dried beans, grains, and seeds can be sprouted. Sprouted beans and grains should be cooked before eating for ease of digestion and best nutrition, while seed sprouts may be enjoyed raw or cooked. Sunflower seed sprouts are delicious and are a good place to start. You can purchase a sprout screen or sprouting lids for mason jars at natural food stores, or make your own by cutting either window screening or the plastic mesh that onions often come bagged in into a square a bit larger than the jar lid; you will secure it to the top of the jar using the ring part of the lid. If you really get serious about sprouting, commercially available sprouters allow you to make larger quantities.

Makes about 1½ cups of sprouts

½ cup beans, grains, or seeds

Rinse the beans, grains, or seeds and place them in a widemouthed 1-quart mason jar. Fill the jar with water and allow it to soak overnight. Place a sprout screen or square of mesh over the jar opening. Drain the water off. Rest the jar in a bowl at an angle so it will drain. Rinse twice daily or more often with cool, fresh water and allow to drain. Sprouts will be ready in 2 to 10 days, depending on the size you want and the sprouting time of the beans, seeds, or grains you're using.

When the sprouts have reached the length you desire, rinse off the hulls, if present, by immersing the sprouts in water and draining, and then drying thoroughly in a salad spinner or on paper towels. If you aren't going to use your sprouts immediately, refrigerate them in a covered container. Most sprouts will keep up to a week refrigerated.

Sprouted Lentil Salad

Lentils were one of the first foods to be cultivated, for good reason. They are high in fiber, folate, and antioxidants, and they cook up quickly. Among the most digestible of the legumes, lentils become even tastier and more digestible when spouted. This versatile dish keeps well and makes a great brown-bag lunch. If your radishes are very fresh and their leaves tender, they will make a delicious, spicy addition to the salad along with the other greens. Sprout a double batch of lentils and turn the rest into lentil soup by simmering them in Bone Broth (chapter 5) or Poultry Stock (chapter 4).

Serves 4 to 6

1 cup green, brown, or black lentils, sprouted for 3 days (see page 56; about 4 cups)

¼ teaspoon sea salt

2 bay leaves

¼ cup Basic Vinaigrette (page 58)

½ cup chopped parsley or cilantro, or a combination

2 cups fresh seasonal salad greens, such as radicchio and arugula

1 bunch radishes, sliced thinly, or 1 watermelon daikon, cut into thin strips

½ cup sprouted sunflower seeds (optional)

Crumbly cheese, such as chèvre or feta, for garnish (optional)

Place the lentils and salt in a medium saucepan and add water to cover by ¼ inch. Cover and place over medium-high heat. When the lentils come to a boil, reduce the heat and simmer, covered, for 12 to 15 minutes, until tender but still firm. Drain but do not rinse.

Add three-quarters of the vinaigrette to the lentils, along with the parsley or cilantro, and gently combine. To serve, arrange the salad greens on a plate and mound the lentils on top. Garnish with the radishes, sunflower seeds, and cheese, and drizzle the remaining vinaigrette over all.

Basic Vinaigrette

The two types of raw vinegar in this vinaigrette contribute beneficial enzymes that aid digestion. I prefer dressings with a lot of zing—if you don't, increase the proportion of oil to vinegar. Making your own salad dressing is so easy and the results are so much tastier than any dressing you'll buy at the store that once you're in the habit of making it, you'll never go back to store-bought. You can find umeboshi plum vinegar, a product of natural fermentation, at health food stores and Asian markets. If you can't find it, omit it and add ¼ teaspoon of sea salt to the dressing. Another way to give the dressing a probiotic kick is to use whey or pickle brine for part of the vinegar.

Makes about ½ cup

- 1 teaspoon prepared mustard
- 2 tablespoons apple cider vinegar
- ½ teaspoon umeboshi plum vinegar
- 1 teaspoon dried or chopped fresh herbs, such as oregano, tarragon, or herbes de Provence
- ¼ cup organic extra-virgin olive oil, cold-pressed walnut oil, or a combination

Put the mustard into a small glass jar with a lid. Add the vinegars and herbs, and shake briskly to combine. Add the olive oil to the jar and shake briskly until the dressing is emulsified.

Variations

- Add ½ teaspoon of chopped capers or anchovies, 2 tablespoons of crumbled blue cheese or crème fraîche, or 1 teaspoon of minced green garlic.

- For Caesar-style dressing, omit the umeboshi vinegar and herbs and add 1 raw pastured or organic egg yolk, the juice of 1 lemon, 1 tablespoon of finely grated Parmesan cheese, and 2 anchovy fillets, and blend with an immersion blender or in a food processor until smooth.

Kale Caesar Salad

Using kale instead of romaine lettuce gives this old standby a nutritional and flavor boost. The easy-to-grow Lacinato variety, also known as dinosaur kale because of its hidelike texture, gives a tender bite in this dish. Unlike lettuce salads, this one keeps well for a day or two.

Serves 4 to 6

1 bunch kale

½ **cup Caesar-style dressing (see Basic Vinaigrette variations, on the previous page)**

¼ **cup shaved or grated Parmesan cheese**

Pepper

Wash the kale and strip the leaves off of their tough stems. Arrange the leaves in a pile on a cutting board and chop into ¼-inch-wide strips. Place the kale in a large salad bowl and add the dressing. Combine thoroughly and let it sit for an hour or more to soften the kale. Just before serving, toss in the cheese and top with freshly ground pepper.

Lamb Koftas

Lamb is nutrient rich—a good source of beneficial omega-3 fatty acids, selenium, and vitamin B12. Most lamb in markets is pasture-raised, but check with your butcher to be sure. Lamb is considered very warming in Chinese nutrition, and this dish is just the thing to put a spring in your step. Koftas, which are of Middle Eastern origin, make use of inexpensive ground lamb, and are a great way to introduce the lamb-timid to this delicious meat. You can grill the koftas like kebabs, but broiling works as well, and it minimizes the creation of cancer-causing compounds (see chapter 4). Serve it as a first course or light main dish with yogurt or Yogurt Cheese and/or Herb Pesto (both earlier in this chapter). Sprouted Lentil Salad (earlier in this chapter), or sprouted whole wheat pita bread with Sprouted Hummus (chapter 3), would make a great accompaniment.

Serves 3 or 4

1 pound ground lamb

3 cloves minced garlic, or 3 tablespoons finely chopped green garlic, white and green parts

¼ cup finely chopped green onion, white and green parts

¼ cup chopped parsley, cilantro, or a combination

2 teaspoons Spanish smoked paprika

1 teaspoon ground cumin

1 teaspoon cinnamon

½ teaspoon dried rosemary or 1 teaspoon minced fresh rosemary

1 teaspoon salt or 1 teaspoon minced anchovies

1 egg yolk, lightly beaten

Put all the ingredients in a large bowl and mix them well with your clean hands until well combined. Shape the mixture into oblong sausage shapes, one for each person you are serving. Broil (or grill) for 3 or more minutes on each side, until lightly browned but still rare in the center to preserve nutrients.

Note: Don't be afraid to try this recipe with anchovies. Anchovies and lamb are a great combination. No one will know there is fish in the dish, but they will comment on the exceptional flavor. You'll be adding wonderful nutritional benefits along with these small fish (see chapter 5).

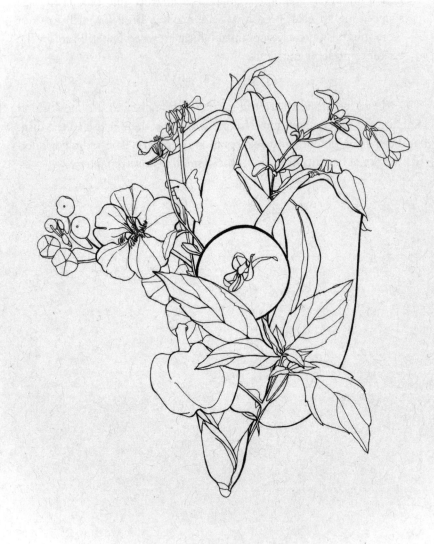

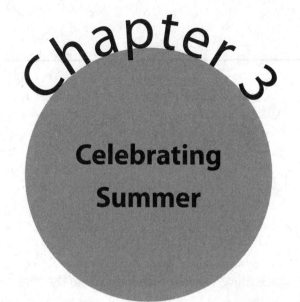

Chapter 3

Celebrating Summer

Chinese medicine teaches that summer is the most yang time of the year. When the days are at their longest, it is natural for us to be busier, and it's okay to sleep less. If you have lived and eaten well in the springtime, clearing away any stagnation left from the winter months, you can harness the energy peak available now for work and play. If you don't have quite enough energy to meet the demands of the long days, or if you are feeling restless or anxious, adjusting your diet can help. Choosing local, seasonal produce attunes your body to the summertime. Five element theory associates the summer with the fire element, the heart organ, the color red, the bitter taste, the emotion of joy, and the sound of laughter. This chapter will explore summer's foods and cooking styles, and consider ancient perspectives and modern nutritional advice for living and eating in the spirit of the season—and for keeping your heart healthy.

At the Market: The Fruits of Summer

The farmers' market in summer is the largest and busiest of the year. Each week, new varieties of summer produce tempt you: wander the aisles languidly; drink in the bright, warm hues of the season; sample everything; and indulge in fresh berries, stone fruits—such as plums, apricots, cherries, peaches, and nectarines—and figs, melons, and the year's first apple varieties. The vegetable array is dizzying: celebrate the return of summer's darlings, such as sweet corn, green beans, basil, summer squash, garlic, okra, cucumbers, avocados, tomatillos, and the season's first blushing local tomatoes. Many crops consumed year-round, such as onions, garlic, and new potatoes, are harvested in summer, and reach a flavor peak now.

Herbs are reaching their maximum growth in the long days, and it is a great time to indulge in bunches of fresh herbs from the market or your garden, seasoning your food generously and drying what you don't use now to bring flavor and nutrition to the cooler seasons. Edible flowers, too, seem to epitomize summer. Enjoy the blooms of borage, calendula, nasturtiums, pansies, roses, and more, and sample the flowers of culinary herbs—most are delicious! The uplifting and antidepressant qualities of flowers are recognized in herbal traditions worldwide and can help attune you to the joy of the season. The energy of the plant world is in fruiting and flowering, and many summer crops are harvested in the form of young, thin-skinned fruits, such as cucumber and summer squash, which are high in water and help to cool and hydrate the body.

As summer progresses, the nightshade family of vegetables, including tomatoes, eggplants, and a dizzying array of peppers, come to market, coinciding with the warmest weather. These vegetables, in part due to their content of slightly toxic *glycoalkaloids*, are considered very cooling to the body and so are best eaten primarily when the weather, or your condition, is hot. Macrobiotics and other holistic nutrition theories caution against the overconsumption of nightshade vegetables, a mainstay in the American diet, on the basis that their glycoalkaloids can disturb calcium metabolism and play a role in joint pain and even arthritis (Colbin 2009). Following a seasonal eating pattern will naturally moderate your intake of nightshades if you focus on eating them around the time of harvest, when their cooling action is most beneficial. If you choose to preserve some of the abundance of the summer foods, methods such as sun-drying tomatoes and peppers, roasting them before freezing, home canning, and fermentation all tend to counterbalance the cooling effects of these vegetables, making them appropriate to eat in cooler seasons.

Cooking, and Not Cooking, in the Summertime

The abundance of the summer harvest reminds us that the summer diet is naturally the most diverse of the year. Strive to sample as much of the variety of summer produce as you can. Fruits and vegetables can make up the bulk of your diet in summertime; in the warm seasons you can think of grains, beans, and animal products more as condiments. The most suitable cooking styles for summer are quick and light. Techniques such as sautéing, stir-frying, steaming, and fermenting for short periods, as well as *not* cooking—that is, eating foods raw—are all in harmony with this season and with your need to minimize both the time spent in the kitchen and your use of the oven. It's also a great time to experiment with *hypercooking*, or selecting dishes that require a minimum of heating time. If you are using a cast-iron skillet, for example, turn off the heat before a dish is done, cover it, and use residual heat to finish the cooking.

Consider carefully the role of raw foods in your diet. Chinese medicine has traditionally warned against consuming too much cold and raw food, which is said to be weakening to the digestive system and the spleen. Some portion of this concern no doubt stems from the context in which Chinese medicine evolved: the vast majority of people were subsistence farmers, and there were very real concerns about sanitation. The ancient admonishment against eating raw food offered protection against food-borne illness. Chinese medicine identifies raw food as cleansing and cooling, which may be undesirable for undernourished people but is often desirable for overnourished people, such as the vast majority of Americans today. In modern North America, improved sanitation has reduced the risk of pathogens carried by water, but problematic factory-farming practices continue to threaten the safety of the food supply and pose a potential threat to eaters of raw foods. Consider the disturbing thought that the strain of *E. coli* that sickened many eaters of prewashed bagged spinach in 2006 is one that exists primarily in grain-fed feedlot cattle (Maki 2006).

While no traditional diet depended solely on raw foods—even in tropical climates, people consume mostly cooked foods—most include some raw foods, particularly raw fermented foods. Raw animal products are eaten almost universally in traditional diets (Fallon 2000). Before you say "yuck" to the idea of raw animal foods, remember the concentrated flavor of real Parmesan cheese, the tender bite of a good ceviche, or the voluptuousness of steak tartare. Raw animal foods, in particular, are concentrated sources of vitamin B6 and detoxifying glutathione, both of which are destroyed by cooking.

The best way to ensure the safety of raw animal foods is to know your producer. I avoid eating factory-farmed beef and lamb raw, but enjoy pastured or organic beef and lamb raw when I source it from a farmer I know and trust. According to the USDA, freezing beef or lamb for fourteen days and then thawing it will effectively kill any parasites that might be present. Raw pork and chicken are best avoided due to the chance of contamination. While fish can contain parasites, the time-honored method of preparing raw fish by marinating it in an acidic medium, used in making ceviche and Hawaiian *poke*, serves to kill pathogens. So, too, does the practice of serving sushi and sashimi with detoxifying herbs such as shiso leaf and pickled ginger.

Most people will do well eating more raw food during the long days of summer, as their cooling and detoxifying effect is needed. Those who enjoy strong digestion can eat over half of their foods raw in the summertime. If you are prone to digestive challenges, such as bloating and loose stools, or if you tend to feel cold easily, you will do best with less raw food but may eat more traditionally fermented foods, like sauerkraut and pickles, yogurt, buttermilk and crème fraîche, kombucha, kefir, and miso.

Grilling is a popular summer cooking style in North America, while in Asia grilling and barbequing are considered very warming methods and are practiced more often in the colder seasons. While the primal taste of grilled meat is a human pleasure not to be denied, cooking over a smoky fire tends to create carcinogenic compounds in meat (but not vegetables), in particular heterocyclic amines. Marinating meat before grilling—in marinades that contain antioxidants, such as red wine, wine vinegar, garlic, olive oil, citrus juice and zest, and culinary herbs, especially parsley, cilantro, and rosemary—has been shown to negate or greatly reduce the production of these harmful compounds (Smith et al. 2008), and serving grilled meat with condiments full of spices and fresh herbs, such as those that follow in chapter 5, will provide your body with antioxidant protection to counter any ill effects of this cooking style.

The Heart in Chinese Medicine

The heart is the most important of the internal organs and is called the emperor organ in Chinese medicine. Not only does the heart govern the circulation of blood throughout the body, but it is also said to house the mind, which includes the intellect, the emotions, the consciousness, and the spirit. The health of your heart shows in the vibrancy of your complexion, while the vitality of your spirit is said to be reflected in your eyes. The connection between the eyes and the spirit is made the world over; think of the saying, "The eyes are the windows to the soul." It is striking to note that in traditional Chinese medical theory, the functions that are ascribed to the brain in the West are located in the heart. The ancient texts recognized the anatomical brain, but it was not considered a particularly important organ. Modern Chinese medicine, of course, incorporates the insights of Western science on the function of the brain. Yet the traditional conception of the heart as the mental and emotional center remains. Contemporary research, particularly in the field of psychoneuroimmunology, is bringing forth new information and new connections that support the ancient Chinese mind-body-spirit link (Pearsall 1998), connecting psychological and physical health.

Poor diet, overwork, weakness in the other organs, and emotional stress are the most common causes of imbalances in heart energy. Excesses of any emotion, even positive emotions such as excitement, can in time lead to damage to the heart. The traditional Chinese conception of a healthy emotional life is one in which you experience all of the emotions, yet they are always flowing and never in excess. Getting stuck in any one emotion for too long can cause damage to the organ associated with that emotion and eventually lead to damage to the heart, the master organ of your emotional life.

If the heart energy is weakened by stress, overwork, or emotional trauma, symptoms such as palpitations (a feeling that the heart is racing or beating irregularly), shortness of breath, low energy, dizziness, anxiety, poor memory, and excessive dreaming may result. Chinese medicine teaches that the heart governs the blood and that the mind is housed in the blood, so when the blood is weak, the heart is affected, and the mind is not well rooted and becomes restless, overactive, and ungrounded. Deficient blood can lead to a scattered, chattering mind, which may spill over from night into day, causing insomnia. To build your blood, first strengthen the digestion following the suggestions in chapter 1. Certain foods help to enrich the blood, calm the spirit, and settle anxiety. Many of them are iron-rich foods that treat anemia and improve the red blood cells' oxygen-carrying capacity. They include beef, lamb, mussels, oysters, liver, egg yolks, dark leafy greens (except spinach and chard), sprouts, sea vegetables, beans (especially those that are dark in color), whole grains, dark fruits such as berries, grapes, and plums, and dried fruit. To assist in the absorption of iron from nonanimal foods, be sure to consume them with foods rich in vitamin C, such as fresh fruits and vegetables.

Chinese nutrition also teaches that eating heart can directly nourish that organ. Heart is lean muscle tissue, high in iron and the densest food source of *coenzyme Q10* (CoQ10), an important nutrient for the heart muscle, now used therapeutically to treat heart disease (Sinatra 2005). Heart meat lacks the strong flavor of other organ meats, and ground heart can be easily incorporated into burgers, meat loaf, and other ground meat dishes for a thrifty source of heart-strengthening nutrition. A popular Peruvian dish, *anticuchos*, consists of cubed beef heart marinated in olive oil and vinegar and grilled.

While the heart is generally protected from external pathogenic factors (which attack the organ that constitutes a protective membrane around the heart, the pericardium), it can be damaged from within by a buildup of *internal heat*. The Chinese concept of internal heat parallels the Western understanding of inflammation. Acute inflammation is the familiar process that occurs in your body when you have an injury. It is characterized by swelling, redness, warmth, and pain, and is used by the body to isolate and begin to fight infection or injury. In Chinese medicine, this state is termed *excess heat* or *full heat*. Chronic inflammation can develop if acute inflammation is incompletely resolved or if insults to the body are continuous, resulting in overactive immune and inflammatory responses. Chinese medicine describes long-term, low-grade inflammation as *deficient* or *empty heat*. If the heart is damaged by excess heat, such symptoms as palpitations, thirst, ulcers of the mouth and tongue, insomnia or sleep disturbed by excessive dreaming, feeling hot and agitated, and a bitter taste in the mouth after a bad night's sleep may result, whereas the more insidious symptoms of deficient heat include palpitations, insomnia, poor memory, anxiety, uneasiness, night sweats, and a dry mouth and throat (Maciocia 1989). Interestingly, Western science is increasingly linking heart and cardiovascular disease to inflammatory conditions, echoing the insights of the ancient Chinese.

The flavor associated with the summer season is bitter, and this flavor is said to be strengthening to the heart. The bitter flavor aids digestion, stimulating the release of bile and supporting the assimilation and metabolism of the fats you eat. Bitter foods exert a cooling effect on the body, allowing us to adapt to the summer heat, and may also help in reducing inflammation. Choose more bitter foods if you are feeling overheated or mentally scattered. Bitter foods available in the summertime include amaranth, corn, quinoa, red lentils, bitter greens (particularly those in the *Brassica* family, including kale, collards, arugula, and mustard greens), green onions, chives, okra, sesame seeds, sunflower seeds, pistachios, and almonds.

Many of the potentially addictive, consciousness-altering substances we commonly consume are classified as having a bitter flavor in Chinese medicine, including coffee, tea, chocolate, liquor, beer, wine, and tobacco, no doubt reflecting an ancient understanding of their powerful effects on the heart-mind. Eating the above foods with a bitter flavor can help calm cravings for excesses of the mind-altering foods and drugs, and serving bitter foods, especially greens, with meals can reduce the urge for the after-meal coffee and cigarette.

The Heart in Western Medicine

The heart and cardiovascular system are responsible for blood circulation, which distributes oxygen, nutrients, fluids, and hormones throughout the body, removes waste products, contributes to the infrastructure of the immune system, and regulates body temperature (Aaronson and Ward 2007). The smooth functioning of this system is therefore critical not only to optimal energy but also to life itself. Heart disease has been the number one killer in North America for over eighty years, and rates are increasing worldwide (Libby et al. 2002). Our look at the relationship between nutrition and heart health necessarily begins with an evaluation of the vast public health experiment conducted in the United States for the past fifty years.

Decades of Dietary Advice: The Lipid Hypothesis

Americans have been told since the 1950s by the government, nutritionists, public health experts, the media, and the food industry to reduce the fat content of our diets, substitute vegetable fat for animal fat, and reduce our cholesterol intake. This massive experiment was based on a hypothesis known as the *lipid hypothesis*, which held that fat and cholesterol in the diet raise cholesterol levels in the blood, promoting atherosclerosis, or the buildup of lesions in the walls of the arteries, which inhibits circulation and is linked to the various types of cardiovascular disease. To reduce our risk of heart disease, Americans were told to eat less fat, especially saturated fat, and cholesterol.

And we listened: we changed our diets. According to the National Health and Nutrition Intake survey undertaken in 2004, from 1971 to 2000 fat intake, especially saturated fat intake, has gone down as a percentage of calories (Hu et al. 2001); however, *total* calorie intake has gone up, reflecting an increase in carbohydrate consumption, particularly consumption of refined carbohydrate foods and drinks (Gross et al. 2004). Death rates from heart disease have gone down, but this is mostly attributed to improvements in coronary care, as the rate of hospital admissions for a first heart attack has been stable (Rosamond et al. 1998). The actual *incidence* of heart disease has changed little, if at all (Taubes 2007). Furthermore, the twin epidemics of diabetes and obesity (combined in the now widely used term *diabesity*) have increased each decade of the experiment (Mokdad et al. 2001). The low-fat diet advice doesn't seem to be working.

In 1977, public health recommendations for the US population were to reduce fat intake to less than 30 percent. The resulting shift to a diet high in refined carbohydrate has since been observed as actually *promoting* atherosclerotic changes and high blood levels of triglycerides, which are linked to heart disease, obesity, and diabetes (German and Dillard 2004). It is now widely acknowledged in the scientific literature that "the low-fat campaign has been based on little scientific evidence and may have caused unintended health consequences" (Hu et al. 2001).

While a sea change is occurring in the science of dietary fat and disease, many sources of nutrition information for the public are lagging behind. Nutrition authorities are just beginning to amend their advice and bring focus to the *types* of fat in the diet rather than the *amount* of fat (ibid). Early versions of this new breed of dietary advice emphasized replacing saturated fat in animal foods with polyunsaturated fat from vegetable sources, although the experimental evidence for such a change was contradictory. In several of the large studies that *did* show a protective effect against heart disease, when this change was found to slightly reduce the chance of death by heart attack, it also tended to be found to increase cancer rates and the chance of death by suicide, violence, or accidents (Golomb 1998), resulting in no change in overall mortality.

A CLOSER LOOK AT CHOLESTEROL

The notion that a high level of cholesterol in the blood is harmful has been under constant revision by the scientific community over the past forty years, if not in the minds of the public and food manufacturers. Let's take a closer look at cholesterol. What exactly is it? Cholesterol is a waxy substance found in most tissues of the body and manufactured by the liver and other body tissues. It is used for tissue repair; for producing testosterone, estrogen, precursors of other hormones, *adrenocorticosteroids* (hormones released by the body under stress), and vitamin D; for creating serotonin receptors; and for producing bile salts. For most people, cholesterol in the diet does not have an appreciable impact on blood cholesterol (Hu et al. 2001). When more cholesterol is consumed, less is produced by the body. In the diet, it is found exclusively in animal products, especially eggs, butter, liver, animal fats, and certain shellfish.

It has been found that total cholesterol measurements have little predictive value for heart disease. By 1977, it was known that while LDL (low-density lipoprotein) cholesterol is a "marginal risk factor" for heart disease, higher HDL (high-density lipoprotein) cholesterol levels actually protect against heart disease (Castelli et al. 1977). These observations have led to the popular characterization of the HDL as the "good cholesterol" and LDL as the "bad cholesterol." HDL cholesterol transports fatty acids from the body to the liver, and LDL cholesterol transports fatty acids from the liver to the body. There has been widespread critique in the scientific community of such a characterization of cholesterol subtypes as "good" and "bad." One researcher observed that "this is like calling an ambulance travelling from the base to the patient a 'bad ambulance,' and the one travelling from the patient back to the base a 'good ambulance'" (Campbell-McBride 2007, 30).

Both the public and the scientific community have often fallen into the trap of confusing association with causality. Cholesterol levels in the body are constantly changing, and tracking their changes *may* tell us something about processes going on in the body that we can use to make prognoses—or not. When LDL is elevated, for example, it may be being transported to the tissues for some reason, most likely because there is tissue damage happening somewhere in the body and the cholesterol is needed for repair. Critics of the lipid hypothesis have suggested that blaming the cholesterol for the damage is like blaming the police because they have been found at the scene of the crime. Science writer Susan Allport (2006, 52) sums it up well: "A truth about serum cholesterol: it was, is, and always will be nothing more than a surrogate marker for heart disease. Half the people with heart disease don't have elevated cholesterol levels. Half the people with elevated cholesterol don't have heart disease."

The last ten years of scientific research on heart disease have increasingly shifted focus from dietary and blood lipids to the processes of both *inflammation* and *oxidative damage* in promoting atherosclerosis (Libby 2002). Inflammation is a healthy response to tissue damage or infection, and is followed by tissue repair and a return to a normal, noninflamed state. However, long-term inflammation can become chronic. *Oxidation* is a chemical processes that occurs constantly in the body, functioning to neutralize unwanted chemicals or foreign particles. Oxidation produces *free radicals*, which are unstable molecules missing an electron in their outer shell. An excess of free radicals beyond what is needed by the body creates a state of oxidative stress, which can cause tissue damage and spur inflammation. Free radicals are neutralized by *antioxidants* made in the body and derived from the diet. Both our levels of oxidative stress and the amount of inflammation in our bodies are strongly influenced by our diets and the dietary fats we consume. Let's take a closer look at the types of fat we eat and their effects.

Dietary Fats and Their Effects

Fat in the diet serves many important functions. Every good cook knows that fat is the carrier of flavor in foods, and when you reduce the fat in a recipe, you must compensate somehow, often by adding a sweetener to provide flavor and moisture. Fat intake, along with protein intake, signals a hormonal response to eating that makes us feel full and satisfied. Fat is vital for many aspects of body structure, creating cell membranes and nerve sheaths, moisturizing the skin and hair, and carrying important fat-soluble vitamins. The following are the types of fat found in food:

- *Saturated fats* are solid at room temperature and consist of carbon chains in which every available site is taken up by a hydrogen atom. This saturation makes the molecules very stable and resistant to oxidative damage, even when used in high-heat cooking. Saturated fats comprise about 50 percent of the fatty acids in most cell membranes in the human body, with higher concentrations in the brain and nervous system. Saturated fats are found in animal foods, ranging from around 40 to 50 percent in beef and pork to 30 to 35 percent in poultry, and in tropical vegetable oils, such as coconut and palm oil, which are around 93 percent and 50 percent saturated, respectively. Some saturated fatty acids have been shown to raise both LDL and HDL, while others raise only HDL, leaving LDL unchanged. It has been found, repeatedly, that "dietary intervention by lowering saturated fat intake does not lower the incidence of nonfatal CAD [coronary artery disease]; nor does such dietary intervention lower coronary disease or total mortality" (German and Dillard 2004), although saturated fat continues to be demonized in the popular press and by the food industry.

- *Monounsaturated fats* are unsaturated fats with one double bond, leaving a single site unoccupied by hydrogen ions. This makes them relatively shelf-stable and resistant to oxidative damage in manufacture, storage, and cooking. They are found in nut and seed oils, especially olive oil (75 percent), and in animal foods such as beef (40 to 55 percent) and lard (48 percent). When eaten, they tend to raise HDL and lower LDL, giving rise to their reputation as "heart healthy" oils. They are stable and comparatively resistant to rancidity.

- *Trans fats* are polyunsaturated fatty acids that have been altered by heating or chemical processing to make them behave like saturated fats. Small amounts occur naturally; however, the vast majority enter the diet through the breakdown of unsaturated fats in cooking or the chemical processing used to create solid fats such as shortening or margarine. They tend to raise LDL and lower HDL. A 2008 study showed that naturally occurring trans fats did not lower HDL, however (Chardigny et al. 2008). Trans fats have been shown in numerous studies to raise triglycerides (which are independently associated with an increased risk of heart disease) and increase insulin resistance (Hu et al. 2001), and have been repeatedly associated with cancer and other degenerative diseases. The FDA has determined that there is no safe level of trans fats in the diet, yet they are still present in many processed foods.

- *Polyunsaturated fats* are unsaturated fatty acids containing more than one double bond and, thus, more than one site unoccupied by hydrogen ions. When eaten, they tend to lower LDL, and some also lower HDL. They are found in liquid vegetable oils and many plant and animal foods. They are relatively unstable and subject to oxidation from damage by light, heat, and chemical processing.

- *Essential fatty acids (EFAs)* are unsaturated fatty acids that must be obtained from the diet as they cannot be made by the body. The two major types are linoleic acid (a polyunsaturated fatty acid with a double bond at the omega-6 position) and alpha-linolenic acid (a polyunsaturated fatty acid with a double bond at the omega-3 position). The myriad functions of the EFAs are largely derived from their conversion into prostaglandins, which play an important role in the regulation of allergies, blood clotting and pressure, gastrointestinal function, heart function, inflammatory response, kidney function, nerve function, and hormone synthesis. Omega-6 fatty acids tend to be converted into pro-inflammatory prostaglandins, while omega-3 fatty acids are converted to anti-inflammatory prostaglandins.

There has been tremendous interest in the essential fats among the scientific community in recent years, and researchers have proposed that a disruption in the ratio of omega-6 to omega-3 fatty acids is behind the increasing rates of chronic disease in modern times. Too much omega-6 in relation to omega-3 is pro-inflammatory and has been linked to "not just heart disease, cancers, depression, immune disorders, and arthritis, but also obesity and diabetes" (Allport 2006, 119). Contemporary American diets often represent a ratio of omega-6 to omega-3 of anywhere from 20:1 to 40:1. Nutritionists recommend a ratio closer to 4:1 or even 2:1, and supplementing therapeutically at 1:1 (Erasmus 2007). Attending to the ratio of fatty acids in your diet may well be of far more importance than modifying the amount of fat, and is one way you can adjust your diet to reduce your risk of inflammation, which can help keep your heart and cardiovascular system healthy (Pollan 2008).

CHOOSING THE HEALTHIEST FATS

When deciding which fats to eat, it is very important to consider the issue of rancidity. Rancid, or oxidized, oil smells bad, fishy, or chemical-like. It is full of free radicals, molecules containing unpaired electrons that can damage cells and DNA, causing *oxidative stress* if not balanced by antioxidants. Oxidative stress is the culprit in many signs of aging, such as wrinkles and gray hair. It comes from many sources: it is the total burden placed on living things by the activity of free radicals, which are created by both normal metabolism and environmental exposures to toxins, such as tobacco smoke. Free radicals are also consumed in the diet, as when you eat rancid fats. As Andrew Weil (2005, 76) puts it, "a good case can be made that health depends on a balance between oxidative stress and anti-oxidant defenses." Most commercially available vegetable oils and many fish oils are already rancid because they have been produced by solvent extraction, a process that uses both high heat and chemicals to extract the oils of seeds or beans. They don't smell bad because further chemicals are added to cover up the off smells. Even high omega-3 oils such as soybean and canola, touted for their health benefits by manufacturers, are largely already rancid in the commercial trade.

When you seek to balance the ratio of omega-3 and omega-6 fatty acids in the diet, it is important to be mindful of obtaining these fatty acids with a minimum of oxidation. For both types of fatty acids, consuming them in their original form—embedded in whole foods—will help ensure that they are not oxidized. Seek out liquid vegetable oils processed without heat or chemicals (which will be labeled "expeller-pressed"), and store them protected from heat and light (Erasmus 2007).

Cold-pressed flaxseed and hempseed oils and fish oils sold refrigerated in opaque bottles are popular supplements. They can be sources of undamaged omega-3s only when they are very fresh, though there is increasing evidence that these oils are so volatile that consuming them in excess may actually increase oxidative stress (Masterjohn 2010). Rather than choosing fish oil and other supplements, a traditional nutritional approach encourages getting your omega-3 fatty acids from eating a variety of sustainably sourced fish and seafood, dairy products, and the fats and flesh of pastured animals. In addition, leafy greens (especially wild greens and seaweeds), walnuts, and flaxseeds are sources of omega-3 fats, albeit in smaller amounts than animal sources (Simopoulos 1998). Ironically, while omega-3 fatty acids are the most abundant fatty acids on earth (as they are the primary fatty acid in growing green plants), they are easily damaged and have become scarce in the modern food supply (Crawford et al. 2000; Pollan 2008). Many of the benefits of omega-3s are blocked by an excess of omega-6 fatty acids, which tend to promote inflammation. Minimizing your intake of corn, soy, cottonseed, and nonoleic safflower and sunflower oils and factory-farmed animal foods will help ensure a healthy ratio of omega-3 to omega-6 fatty acids in your system.

Animal foods from animals raised on pasture will contain a higher ratio of omega-3 fatty acids, as these are the fatty acids in grass. When animals are raised or finished in confined animal feeding operations (CAFOs, or feedlots), their grain-based diet shifts the fatty-acid ratio from omega-3 to omega-6 (ibid). This is yet another reason to seek out animal foods from small, pasture-based farms, which also serve to protect the environment and encourage carbon sequestration. When you buy dairy foods from pastured cows, choose full-fat, ideally nonhomogenized, dairy products for the highest concentration of beneficial, undamaged essential fats. When dairy processors remove fat from dairy products, they generally add nonfat dry milk powder (check your labels), which is a source of potentially dangerous oxidized cholesterol.

Virgin and extra-virgin olive oil are two of the few oils found in supermarkets that are mechanically processed at low heat. You'll need to go to a health food or specialty market to find vegetable oils that are expeller-processed. Store them tightly sealed and away from light to protect them from rancidity. Heating fats and oils naturally causes some damage to them through oxidization. Saturated fats are more resistant to heat damage. That is why butter, ghee, lard, tallow, and chicken and duck fat have been used for frying in many cultures. While lard is a versatile fat for cooking that can withstand high heat and that has a mild, neutral flavor, you'll need to make a point of finding natural lard from pastured animals, as the lard available in most supermarkets contains artificial hydrogenated oils. Liquid vegetable oils are best consumed raw and unheated, in salad dressings and sauces, to gain the maximum benefit of their essential fatty acids. Olive oil, *high-oleic* safflower oil, and high-oleic sunflower oil (from seeds bred to increase their content of monounsaturated fats, or oleic acids), and coconut and palm kernel oils are the most stable of the vegetable fats to use in cooking and baking. The following chart summarizes the best sources of fats and oils to protect the health of your heart.

Instead of...	Choose...
Margarine, "healthy spreads"	Butter, olive oil, or expeller-pressed walnut oil for dipping bread
Vegetable shortening, shelf-stable lard	Pastured lard, coconut oil, ghee, duck fat, bacon grease
Vegetable oil	Virgin or extra-virgin olive oil, high-oleic safflower or sunflower oil, coconut oil, pastured lard, duck fat, ghee
Commercial salad dressing	Homemade dressings made with healthful fats
Low-fat or nonfat dairy products	Full-fat, nonhomogenized ("cream-top"), or raw milk and dairy

EATING AND DRINKING AGAINST OXIDATIVE STRESS

How do you protect yourself against oxidative stress? Because oxidative stress is a side effect of the body's detoxification efforts, you can minimize drug, chemical, and toxin exposure in general and in the diet in particular using the strategies outlined in chapter 2: avoid consuming rancid oils (including all partially hydrogenated vegetable oils, commercial chemically processed oils, oils that have been heated too high, and fats in most packaged and processed foods), and seek out sources of antioxidants in your diet. Many of the seasonal foods of summer are very high in antioxidants, in part because plants use antioxidants to protect their flowers and fruits (and their DNA) from oxidative damage, which occurs more in the long, sunny days of summer. What are the best food sources of antioxidants? Berries are a well-known source, particularly strawberries and blueberries, but the less glamorous plum is an even richer source of antioxidants, and so are apples and dried beans, especially those that are dark in color. Most herbs and spices are extremely high in antioxidants, and the category of culinary herbs ranks behind only medicinal herbs in antioxidant power (Carlsen et al. 2011). Culinary amounts of herbs and spices—that is, one half to one teaspoon of many common seasonings—have been found to have a greater amount of antioxidants than average servings of fruits and vegetables (Dragland et al. 2003).

Other year-round foods that confer antioxidant protection include those rich in vitamin E, the premier antioxidant of the oils, found in fresh nuts and seeds and their cold-pressed oils, freshly ground wheat, and animal products from animals fed their whole lives on grass. While black, white, and green teas have received much press for their high antioxidant content and health value, coffee is the number one source of antioxidants in the American diet (Svilaas et al. 2004). Tea, chocolate, and red wine all make significant contributions, too. If you drink coffee and tea, be sure to choose organic to avoid pesticide exposure, and grind coffee fresh to maximize the antioxidant content. Red wine has received a lot of press for its high antioxidant content, which varies by variety. Moderate alcohol consumption seems to confer protection from heart disease (Yusuf et al. 2004). Why not just take your antioxidants in supplement form? The preponderance of research on the topic has shown that the antioxidants are best obtained from whole foods, not supplements, and that supplemental antioxidants actually increase disease incidence in some cases (Bjelakovic and Gluud 2007).

Nourishing the Heart and Spirit

What is the best way to ensure the health of your heart? The largest comprehensive international study on heart disease to date, known as the INTERHEART study, is a comprehensive case-control study of tens of thousands of people using data from fifty-two countries. The study authors concluded that over 90 percent of heart disease risk is associated with the following modifiable factors: blood lipid abnormalities, smoking, diabetes, hypertension, abdominal obesity, and psychosocial factors, while protective factors included daily consumption of vegetables and fruit, regular exercise, and moderate alcohol intake (Yusuf et al. 2004). The "psychosocial factors" included work, home, and financial stress; depression; and stressful life events, which were found to have a significant impact on the risk of heart disease for all people regardless of region or gender (Rosengren et al. 2004). Thus, this study concluded that nearly all of the risk of heart disease can be eliminated with diet and lifestyle changes, rather than medication or medical intervention.

The INTERHEART study findings echo the insights of Chinese medicine linking the health of the heart to the health of our emotional lives. In his sixteenth-century treatise on healing, Korean doctor Hur Jun (quoted in Fruehauf 2011) penned the following advice to traditional doctors, advice that we all would do well to apply to our own self-healing.

> If you wish to bring about real healing, you must first and foremost treat a person's heart.... You must get it to a place where it can safely abandon all doubting and worrying and obsessing in endlessly looping patterns, where it can let go of any anxiety provoking imbalances, and where it is willing to surrender all "me, me, me" and all "this is his/her fault!" Try and awaken the heart to acknowledge and regret all the wrong that one has done, to lay down all selfish attachments, and to transform one's small and self-centered world for the glorious universe in which we are all one, and wherein there is nothing to do but praise its existence.

This is the master method of the enlightened physician—healing through the heart.

Seeking lifestyles and practices that nourish the body, mind, and spirit will help you find a true path to vitality and relaxed energy, the gift of a strong and healthy heart.

Summer Recipes

To attune yourself to the energy of summer, begin incorporating more spicy, pungent foods into your diet. Hot spices such as garlic, chiles, horse-radish, and ginger can help bring your body's energy to the surface, dispersing heat. Traditional cuisines of very hot and humid climates, such as Southeast Asia and parts of India and China, are spicy enough to induce sweating, thereby cooling the body. Iced foods and liquids are generally not eaten in traditional cultures as they are so often in North America. They are considered overcooling, making the body work harder to warm them up to body temperature, and thus encouraging overheating. Instead of reaching for iced foods, choose bitter foods, such as cucumbers with their peels, to gently cool the body. As during the rest of the year, much of the summer diet should be comprised of naturally sweet foods that harmonize and provide energy in the form of carbohydrates.

Summer Shopping List

Animal Products: beef, chicken, lamb, seasonal fish and seafood

Beans: red lentils, red beans, tempeh and tofu, mung beans

Grains: amaranth, corn, quinoa, rice

Vegetables: arugula, sweet corn, green beans, basil, summer squash, garlic, okra, cucumbers, avocados, tomatillos, tomatoes, peppers, eggplant, green onions, chives, cilantro, snow peas, chard, sprouts, mushrooms, watercress, edible flowers

Fruits: apricots, peaches, plums, nectarines, apples, strawberries, blueberries, blackberries, raspberries, melons, citrus

Herbs, Spices, and Condiments: garlic, hot peppers, horseradish, ginger, fresh herbs such as tarragon, rosemary, oregano,

Rosemary Lemonade

Fermenting this favorite summertime refresher adds beneficial probiotics while reducing the amount of sugar it contains. The rosemary and lemon zest add flavor as well as antioxidants. Try this technique with other seasonal herbs, such as mint, rose geranium, or lavender.

Makes 2 quarts

7 cups filtered water

½ cup evaporated cane juice, palm sugar, coconut sugar, or other minimally refined natural sugar

2 tablespoons fresh or dried rosemary

Zest and juice of 3 lemons

1 cup Yogurt Whey (page 49) or Ginger Bug (page 85)

In a large pot, bring the water to a boil, add the evaporated cane juice, and stir to dissolve. Remove the pot from the heat, add the rosemary, and cover. Let it cool until it is the temperature of bathwater. Put the lemon juice, lemon zest, and whey into a 2-quart mason jar. Pour in the sweetened herb water, screw on the lid, and allow it to ferment in a warm place, such as the top of your refrigerator, for 2 days. Watch for small bubbles rising to the top of the jar, indicating that fermentation is taking place. Strain the lemonade into two 1-quart bottles or jars with screw tops—the liquid should come nearly to the tops of the bottles for the best results—cap tightly, and let ferment for 2 days more before storing in the refrigerator. Chill before opening and open cautiously, releasing the carbon dioxide slowly if needed so that the drink doesn't foam out of the bottle. The lemonade will keep, refrigerated, for several weeks.

Hibiscus and Rose Hip Soda

This beautiful red drink, adapted from Jessica Prentice's book *Full Moon Feast*, epitomizes summer, benefits the heart, and is high in vitamin C. Hibiscus tea has been shown in several studies to reduce blood pressure as effectively as medication when consumed regularly (McKay et al. 2011), offering natural and delicious protection for the heart. This soda also gives a hit of probiotics for digestive health. You can find dried hibiscus flowers at herb stores or in Latino markets (sold as jamaica); rose hips are available at herb stores.

Makes 2 quarts

7 cups filtered water

⅔ cup evaporated cane juice or coconut sugar

¼ cup dried hibiscus flowers

1 tablespoon dried rose hips

1 cup Yogurt Whey (page 49) or Ginger Bug (see below)

Put the filtered water in a pot and bring it to a boil. Stir in the evaporated cane juice and turn off the heat. Allow it to cool. Put the hibiscus, rose hips, and whey into a 2-quart mason jar and add the sweetened, cooled water to fill the jar. Screw the lid on the jar and put it in a warm place for 2 days. You will notice small bubbles rising to the top of the jar, indicating that fermentation is taking place.

Strain equal amounts into two 1-quart glass bottles or jars with screw tops (I reuse mineral water bottles); they should be full nearly to the top. Screw the lids on tightly, label and date the bottles, and return them to the warm place for another 2 to 3 days, or until the soda becomes slightly bubbly.

Transfer the bottles to the fridge. Once the soda is cold, you can enjoy it anytime. When you are ready to drink the soda, open the bottles carefully, because they may have built up a lot of carbonation. Turn the lid very slowly to see if the drink begins to release foam. If it does, allow it to release some of the carbon dioxide before opening it more. Ease the lid open bit by bit to release the pressure until it's safe to remove the lid without the drink foaming out of the bottle. This way you won't lose your drink to its carbonation. The soda will keep for several weeks in the refrigerator.

Ginger Bug

Ginger bug is a traditional starter for fermented drinks, and it is easily made. You'll need to start several days before you make the drink. Place 1 cup of filtered water in a pint jar and add 2 teaspoons of freshly grated ginger. Stir in 2 teaspoons of evaporated cane juice, put the lid on, and shake. Store it in a warm place in the kitchen. Each day, add another 2 teaspoons each of grated ginger and evaporated cane juice, and shake to mix. After a few days, look for small bubbles rising to the top of the jar. This can happen in 2 days in hot weather, longer if the weather is cool. For best results, use the bug to brew your drink as soon as the bubbles appear.

Red Lentil Dal with Sweet Corn

In Chinese medicine, red lentils are classified as having a slightly bitter taste, which makes them particularly beneficial to the heart, the organ most important to nourish in the summertime. Dal, a dish of simmered and spiced legumes, is a staple food in India and Nepal, and can be enjoyed for breakfast, lunch, or dinner. It is also traditionally used as the basis of a seasonal fast at the beginning of summer. This recipe can be easily varied by the addition of almost any seasonal vegetable. A bunch of chopped arugula, stirred in during the last few minutes of cooking, is particularly tasty.

Makes 4 to 6 servings

6 cups water

1 cup red lentils, rinsed

One 6-inch strip kombu (see note)

1 tablespoon olive oil or ghee

1 onion, diced small

1 teaspoon mustard seeds

1 tablespoon curry powder or a mixture of 1 teaspoon each of ground cumin, coriander, and turmeric

2 carrots, scrubbed but not peeled and cut in ¼-inch-thick rounds

3 celery stalks, diced

One 1-inch piece unpeeled gingerroot, grated (about 3 tablespoons)

Juice of 1 or 2 lemons

Sea salt

Chopped cilantro, for garnish

Put the water in a large pot and add the lentils; soak overnight if possible. Do not drain, but bring lentils to a boil in their soaking water, lower the heat, and simmer uncovered for 10 minutes, skimming off any foam that rises to the surface. Add the kombu to the pot, cover, and turn the heat down low.

While the lentils are simmering, heat the oil in a skillet; add the onion and sauté for 5 minutes or until it begins to turn translucent. Add the mustard seeds and curry powder, and stir occasionally until the spices give off their fragrance, about 60 seconds. Add the carrots and celery, and continue to cook for a few minutes more, until they begin to brown around the edges. Scrape the vegetables and spices into the pot with the lentils, cover, and simmer until the lentils are soft and creamy, for 10 to 30 minutes more, depending on the age of the lentils.

Take the grated ginger in your hand and squeeze the juice into the pot, or force it through a fine mesh sieve to extract the juice and add it to the pot. Add lemon juice and sea salt to taste. Serve garnished with cilantro.

Note: *Kombu* is a type of seaweed that helps beans cook more quickly and makes them more flavorful and digestible. You can purchase it packaged or in bulk at health and natural food stores.

Sprouted Hummus

If you've cooked dried chickpeas before, you'll be delighted at how much more quickly they cook when you sprout them first. Making this staple spread yourself is empowering, and the results are more digestible—and tastier—than commercial versions. The chickpea miso adds great flavor and is a source of probiotics. Serve with pita, on a sandwich, or as part of a meze platter with grilled lamb or Lamb Koftas (chapter 2).

Makes about 2 cups

1 cup chickpeas, soaked and sprouted for 2 days (see page 56)

Filtered water

One 6-inch strip kombu

2 bay leaves

½ teaspoon sea salt

2 cloves garlic

Juice of 1 lemon

2 tablespoons tahini

1 teaspoon white or chickpea miso

Put the chickpeas in a large pot and cover by about 1 inch with filtered water. Add the kombu and bay leaves, and bring to a boil over medium-high heat. Cover, and reduce the heat to low. Allow the chickpeas to simmer gently until tender, from 1 to 2 hours (or longer), depending on how long the beans have been in storage. When the chickpeas are nearly tender, stir in the salt. Continue cooking until you can easily mash a chickpea against your upper palate with your tongue. Remove from the heat and allow to cool. Remove and discard the bay leaf and kombu, and drain the chickpeas, reserving the liquid.

Place the chickpeas in the bowl of a food processor fitted with the blade attachment, or in a deep bowl. Add the garlic (chop it first if you are mashing by hand), lemon juice, tahini, and miso, and process or mash the mixture into a smooth paste. Add some of the reserved cooking liquid if needed to get a texture you like. The hummus will keep in the refrigerator for up to 2 weeks.

Grass-Fed Steak Tartare

Raw beef is high in vitamin B6, iron, and zinc. The mild taste of the beef is brought out with a balance of spices and ingredients (like anchovies and oil) that add umami, making a heavenly dish that digests easily and is very energizing. If you don't know and trust your beef farmer, ensure that any pathogens are killed by freezing and thawing the meat beforehand. This dish contains a raw egg yolk, so be sure of your egg's origin too. Serve as a first course or light meal with toasted bread, crackers, or lettuce leaves.

Serves 2 as a main course, 4 as a starter

1 pound pastured rib-eye or similar steak, frozen for 14 days and thawed

1 teaspoon Spanish paprika

1 tablespoon rinsed and chopped salt-cured capers

2 tablespoons thinly sliced green onion, white and pale green parts

2 tablespoons minced parsley

1 tablespoon minced shallot

2 tablespoons extra-virgin olive oil

2 tablespoons prepared mustard

2 tablespoons minced, rinsed anchovies

Sea salt

Pepper

1 pastured egg yolk

Remove the bone, if any, from the steak and reserve it for Bone Broth (chapter 5). Chop the steak as finely as possible with a very sharp knife or using a food processor. (If chopping by hand, the chopping will be easier if you chill the meat to just below freezing first.) Mix in the paprika, capers, green onion, parsley, shallot, olive oil, and mustard, and season to taste with sea salt and freshly ground pepper. Mound on a plate and make an indentation in the center. Gently drop the egg yolk into the indentation, garnish with the anchovies, and serve promptly. Each diner can scoop up a bite of beef, egg, and anchovy using bread or lettuce leaves.

Rub for Grilled Lamb

This rub is but one example of a mixture of oil, spices, and seasonings that enhances both the flavor and the nutritional value of grilled meats. Smear it over lamb chops and let it marinate overnight in the refrigerator before grilling. Try it on beef, chicken, or pork as well.

Makes enough for 1 pound of meat

2 cloves garlic

1 tablespoon coarse sea salt

1 tablespoon dried or 2 tablespoons fresh rosemary

½ teaspoon Spanish paprika

½ teaspoon ground cumin

2 tablespoons olive oil

Mash the garlic with a mortar and pestle, and sprinkle in the salt. Continue to mash; as it becomes a paste, add the paprika, cumin, and olive oil, and combine well. Alternatively, combine the ingredients in a food processor and process until they form a coarse paste. Smear it over the meat and let it marinate overnight before grilling.

Green Sauce

This quintessential herb sauce that appears in many cultures has infinite variations. Change the herbs or seasonings, trying anchovies instead of capers, vinegar instead of lemon, or adding some heat with a chile. Serve this with almost any dish, such as scrambled eggs, roasted vegetables, or grilled meats, or atop soup, to add flavor, enzymes, and antioxidant power.

Makes about ⅔ cup

1 tablespoon salt-cured capers

1 shallot or 2 green onions, both green and white parts

1 clove garlic

1 bunch parsley or cilantro, stems removed and reserved for another use

¼ cup leaves of fresh herbs, such as marjoram, basil, dill, tarragon, or thyme

Zest and juice of 1 lemon

½ cup extra-virgin olive oil

Sea salt

Pepper

Soak the capers in water to cover them, while you finely chop together the shallot, garlic, parsley, and herbs. Drain the capers and mince finely. Put the chopped aromatics and capers in a bowl, vigorously stir in the oil until well combined, and season to taste with salt and freshly ground pepper. Alternatively, using a food processor, process the capers, shallot, garlic, parsley, herbs, and lemon together until finely chopped; then slowly drizzle in the olive oil with the motor running until just combined. Season to taste with salt and freshly ground pepper. Serve immediately or store refrigerated for several days.

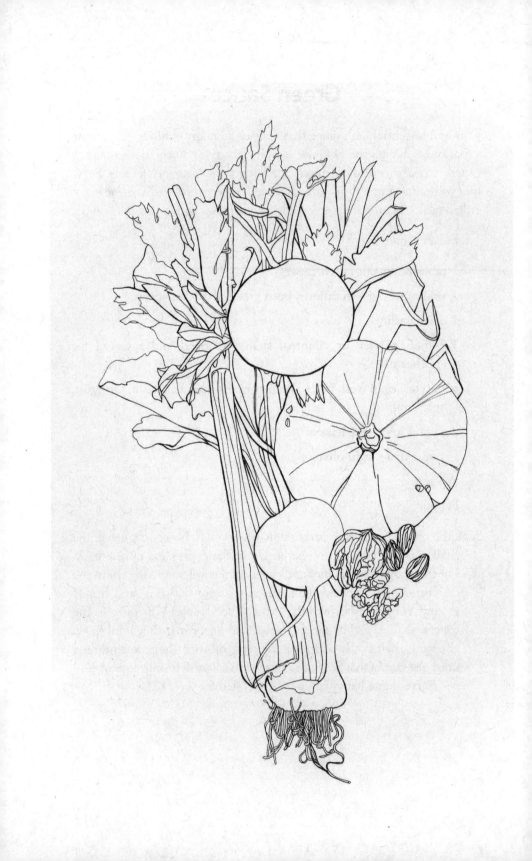

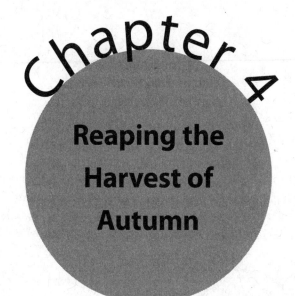

Chapter 4

Reaping the Harvest of Autumn

As the wheel of the seasons turns to fall, the days shorten, the earth cools, and the expanded energy of summer begins to consolidate. It's my favorite time of year at the farmers' market, when the gleaming warm colors of the summer harvest nestle next to the subdued hues of fall. Fall is the season that Chinese medicine associates with the metal element, the lung and large intestine organs, the processes of holding on and letting go, the emotion of grief, the pungent taste, and the color white. The health of your metal element is reflected in the strength of your lungs and immune system, the quality of your skin, and the regularity of your bowels. In the fall, the Chinese classics advise that you should prune away the excess activity of summer like pruning a fruit tree after it bears, consolidate your energy, focus on what is most important, and prepare for the coming of winter.

In this chapter, we'll explore the foods and cooking styles of fall and their many health benefits, with a particular focus on the seasonal foods that strengthen the lungs and large intestine, resulting in increased vitality. We'll connect the ancient Chinese perspective on the physiology of the lungs and large intestine to the modern understanding of the immune system, and explore how proper diet can optimize digestion, immunity, and energy.

At the Market: What's in Season Now

During a stroll through the farmers' market in late September, the last of summer's nightshades, stone fruits, and corn gleam alongside the new arrivals of fall—the rich tones of apples, pears, and pomegranates; autumn-yielding varietals of raspberries and strawberries; the first gold and green winter squashes; sweet potatoes and purple blushing rutabagas; creamy parsnips and other root vegetables of the season. The reappearance of second crops of foods that made their annual debut in the spring—leeks, fennel, green beans, radishes, snap peas, and young turnips and beets—adds to the profusion in many climates. How do you choose?

Thin-skinned, watery summer crops such as nightshade vegetables (see chapter 3), cucumbers, summer squash, and the like tend to have a cooling effect on the body, while the foods harvested later (which take longer to mature on the plant), such as winter squash, and those that grow underground, like root vegetables, tend to be more warming. It is wise to shift the focus of your diet toward these foods as the weather cools, a process that happens naturally when you are a CSA member or gardener, or faithfully stick to crops harvested close to home.

While the advent of refrigeration and industrial agriculture has made meat available year-round, fall is a traditional time for hunting or for slaughtering farm animals, and for preserving this harvest to ensure having enough food in the coming months. As Jessica Prentice writes in her book on seasonal eating by the lunar calendar, *Full Moon Feast* (2006, 209), "In midautumn, when the air is growing colder and the nights longer, comes the Blood Moon...a time when northern dwellers of many cultures would work to ensure that their store of meat would last through the winter." You can echo this rhythm by organizing a whole-animal purchase from a local farm (see resources) to divide up among your friends, stocking your freezer for the winter, or trying your hand at home charcuterie (the art of making preserved meats)—or just get your feet wet with the recipes for preparing a whole duck (pages 00 to 00). The shorter days tend to make pasture-raised eggs less available as fall progresses, so the seasonal eater will naturally reduce egg consumption in these darker months.

Fall Cooking Styles

You'll want to adjust your cooking techniques now to help your body adjust to the shorter, cooler days of fall. Think of cooking foods for longer periods of time, and with a little less water, than in the summer. Traditional Chinese nutrition confirms the cook's instincts, encouraging more baking, sautéing, roasting, stewing, and braising at this time of year, replacing or complementing the raw, steamed, or quickly prepared foods of the warmer seasons. Slower and more complex cooking techniques create rich flavors and meals that warm the body at its core, providing more energy, and are thought by Chinese doctors to help thicken and enrich your blood and body fluids.

The bounty of fall also encourages the art of preserving food, enabling us to capture some of the flavors and nutrients of the harvest to nourish our bodies through the winter. Traditional methods of food preservation, such as drying and fermentation, typically conserve or increase the nutrients and digestibility of food, whereas many modern methods such as industrial canning, ultra-pasteurizing, and the refining of grains tend to decrease them (Fallon 2000). You'll find several recipes for seasonal fermentation projects later in the chapter.

In some climates, spring produce such as beets, turnips, fennel, and snap peas reappear in the fall, reminding us that these two seasons are mirror images of one another. They each entail a transition, moving from balanced day and night at their respective equinoxes to the annual solstices. The produce that matures in these transitional seasons can support our bodies in adjusting to the changing temperatures and light, and in many ways the fall diet is a mirror image of the spring one. Traditional healing systems often advise a fall cleanse, which may be shorter and gentler than a typical spring regimen, to ease the transition into the cooler season. Close to the fall equinox, on September 21 or so, is a good time to do this. While simply choosing seasonal foods will benefit your body, you might want to revisit the spring cleanse described in chapter 2, focusing on the foods and cooking techniques of fall, for a few days to a few weeks at the beginning of each autumn.

Fall Flavors

Chinese nutritional energetics suggests incorporating more sour flavored foods, which have an astringent action, into the diet now to support mental focus and ease the transition to darker days. Seasonal foods like tart apples, late plums, grapes, and leeks, as well as lemons or limes in areas where they grow, and year-round foods like sourdough bread (both wheat and rye), pickles, vinegar, olives, and cultured dairy foods such as yogurt and cheese will help consolidate your body's energy and encourage vitality in the cooler months ahead. Many of these foods are soured by fermentation, adding the potential benefit of probiotics, or live health-promoting bacteria, which I will discuss in detail later in the chapter.

Traditional wisdom encourages the balancing of the contractive action of sour flavors with the expansive, stimulating effects of pungent and mildly spicy flavors. Mildly spicy foods and herbs, such as those listed in chapter 2 for moving liver qi stagnation, will encourage circulation and keep the contraction of fall from becoming too restrictive. If you are having a hard time slowing from the busyness of summer, and need support for mental focus, choose sour flavored foods like those above. On the other hand, if you tend toward winter blues, or are feeling overly sluggish as the season progresses, incorporating more pungent foods, particularly the seasonal ones described next, can help.

The Lungs in Chinese Medicine

The Yellow Emperor's Classic of Medicine (Ni 1995) teaches that autumn is the best time to strengthen or treat imbalances in the lungs. Common sense, too, tells us that autumn brings the onset of the cold and flu season, and it is no accident that fighting off such ailments is one of the functions ascribed to the lungs in Chinese physiology. The lungs are called the "delicate organ" in Chinese, indicating their vulnerability to seasonal pathogens.

The lungs are said to govern respiration, meaning that they extract qi, or oxygen, from the air we breathe and mix it with the nutrients derived from food by the spleen, creating the major source of our daily energy. If your lungs are weak, you may experience fatigue, shortness of breath, or spontaneous sweating. Weak lung energy might also manifest in susceptibility to colds and flu, allergies, asthma, or chronic sinus congestion. The lungs and sinuses, like the digestive tract and the vagina, are uniquely characterized by their lining made of a delicate membrane, the *mucosa*, containing cells that secrete mucus.

Mucus is an important, if underappreciated, body fluid, serving to protect and lubricate tissues, nourish beneficial bacteria and trap harmful ones, and ease the passage of food along the digestive tract. Good health is reflected in the optimal amount and quality of mucus. The body secretes extra mucus in response to pathogens, irritants, or allergens in an attempt to protect itself. Chinese medicine teaches that the while the spleen creates mucus (called *phlegm* when excessive), the lungs store it. In conditions of excess mucus, strengthening the spleen and the digestion (for example, by following the dietary guidelines in chapter 1) is important in healing. Mucous membranes also need sufficient vitamin A to thrive. True vitamin A, called retinol because of its importance to the function of the eyes, is found only in animal foods such as butter, egg yolks, liver, organ meats, and shellfish, particularly when the animals have lived in the wild or grazed on pasture. *Carotenoids*, a group of phytonutrients including beta-carotene, which impart rich colors to plant foods, can, under optimal conditions, be converted into vitamin A by the body (Fallon 2000). This conversion occurs during digestion in the presence of bile, which is released by the gallbladder when a meal including fat is eaten. Hence the wisdom of eating vegetables with olive oil, butter, or cream, which enhances the body's ability to make use of the fat-soluble vitamins they contain.

EATING FOR LUNG HEALTH

The following seasonal and year-round foods are traditional remedies for strengthening the lungs and spleen, and building digestive and respiratory capacity and stamina:

- Whole grains: barley, brown rice, oats, sweet rice (a starchy, short-grained rice)

- Vegetables: carrots, celery, radishes, green beans, mustard greens, onions, olives, pumpkin, yams

- Fruits: apricots, chestnuts, cherries, dates, figs, grapes, pears, raspberries; choose dried fruit or frozen fruit when local fresh fruit is not available

- Nuts: peanuts, walnuts

- Spices: basil, cinnamon, garlic

- Beans: black beans, tofu, tempeh

- Animal foods: beef, duck, eggs, fish, goat milk and cheese, lamb, pork

Pungent and mildly spicy foods can act to stimulate the lungs, break up excessive mucus, and help protect the respiratory system from the effects of airborne pollutants, pathogens, and allergens. Such foods have a long history of traditional use for this purpose, and are being increasingly recognized by science. Dr. Irwin Ziment, a pulmonary specialist, inspired by the finding that Latinos who smoke in the polluted Los Angeles area have a surprisingly low rate of lung cancer, routinely prescribed chiles to his respiratory patients on the basis that they are rich sources of antioxidants and that they contain compounds, common to many spicy tasting herbs, that thin mucus and encourage expectoration (Duke 1997; Pitchford 2002).

In addition to all types of chiles, onion family vegetables such as onions, garlic, leeks, and shallots; the spicier cruciferous vegetables including cabbage, radishes, horseradish, and turnips; and culinary spices such as ginger, wasabi, mustard, and white pepper are considered pungent foods. These are seasonable in the fall and can be eaten regularly to optimize mucus production and movement, and overall lung function. When the problem is not too much mucus but not enough, as when you have a lingering dry cough as you recover from a cold, a traditional Chinese remedy is pears or Asian pears. Try them fresh, poached in apple juice and ginger juice, or puréed with yams in a light bone broth for a nourishing and delicious soup. Other seasonal foods that can soothe a dry cough and moisten dry lungs and sinuses include persimmons, walnuts, carrots, celery, yams, cabbage, watercress, lettuce, peppermint, lemon, and goat's milk.

Fresh nuts are another food harvested in the fall that contains nutrients that are beneficial to the lungs. They are very good sources of vitamin E, which has been linked to protecting the lungs from the effects of air pollution (Packer 1991), and essential fatty acids, as well as cancer-protective, detoxifying ellagic acid (Murray et al. 2005). Look for walnuts, almonds, hazelnuts, pecans, or other nuts that grow in your area. Buy them freshly shelled at the farmers' market or shell them yourself to get the most benefit. Be aware that many commercially packaged nuts are rancid, or have been deep-fried in rancid oils. Simply cooking nuts or, better yet, soaking them overnight before roasting, grinding, or cooking them will make them easier to digest and reduce their load of phytic acid, which can block mineral absorption.

The Large Intestine—and the "Forgotten Organ"

The large intestine is the other internal organ associated with the metal element and the fall season. The function of the large intestine is to move digested food from the small intestine, conduct it downward, reabsorb some of the fluids, and form the stool, which is then excreted. The pairing of the lung and large intestine organs in Chinese medicine reflects an understanding of the body only recently uncovered by Western physiology. They are both lined with mucous membranes and are the home of the majority of our *microbiota*, the bacteria living in and on the human body, which outnumber our own body cells by a factor of ten to one (Lipski 2005). Science is rapidly uncovering the vast importance of these bacteria, 80 percent of which reside in the large intestine, and they have been termed "the forgotten organ" (O'Hara and Shanahan 2006).

YOUR AMAZING MICROBIOTA

Intestinal bacteria perform many functions in your body, such as improving the absorption of nutrients, helping digest lactose (milk sugar) and protein, synthesizing fatty acids and vitamins such as B, K, and A, regulating pH, crowding out potentially harmful bacteria, and regulating the immune system (Lipski 2005). Recent research suggests that having healthy microbiota helps protect you from infections, regulates digestion and metabolism, prevents disease, buffers stress, tames inflammation, and prevents allergies and autoimmune problems (Huffnagle and Wernick 2007). Unfortunately, many factors of modern life, such as the widespread use of antibiotics, a lack of fermented and cultured foods, and the shift in dietary patterns away from whole foods and toward highly refined foods and drinks, contribute to imbalances in digestive flora that are widespread in people today (ibid). Les Dethlefsen observed long-term changes in intestinal bacteria in people from just a single course of antibiotics (Dethlefsen and Relman 2011). Furthermore, modern childbirth and child-rearing practices such as hospital birthing, cesarean sections, lack of or short-term breastfeeding, early vaccination, and frequent antibiotic exposure may interfere with the establishment of healthy intestinal flora from birth (Sachs 2007).

Your diet has a direct impact on your microflora in several ways. When you ingest probiotic foods and beverages such as yogurt, the living bacteria in these foods have immediate beneficial effects as they pass through your gut, and some types even take up temporary residence (Lipski 2005). Archeological evidence suggests that humans have been using fermentation with *lactic acid bacteria* (bacteria that consume carbohydrates and create lactic acid) to preserve food for many thousands of years, and it is posited that the human digestive system evolved around a daily intake of such bacteria (Molin 2001). *Prebiotics* are compounds in food that inhibit the growth of less-friendly bacteria in the gut; they include fiber or certain proteins like *lactoferrin* (found in whey)—both of which encourage the growth of beneficial bacteria—and *phenols*, the most abundant type of antioxidant in plant foods. Finally, *metabiotics* are defined as metabolic by-products of bacterial action that exert beneficial effects. The presence of metabiotics helps explain why even consuming probiotics that are no longer alive, for example, in cooked yogurt and sourdough bread, has beneficial effects on health (Huffnagle and Wernick 2007).

Gary Huffnagle, a highly respected immunologist and microbiologist, suggests in his 2007 book *The Probiotics Revolution* that many people will experience health benefits by adding a wide variety of fermented foods to the diet (ibid.). These benefits include increased energy, resistance to illness, stress reduction, fewer digestive disorders, fewer allergies, and much more. I have observed many patients in my acupuncture practice noticing improved digestion, energy, and health when they began to incorporate a wide variety of fermented foods into their daily diets. Fermented foods are typically easier to digest than their unfermented counterparts. In a sense, they have been predigested, making their nutrients easier to assimilate. However, if you are unaccustomed to eating such foods, it is wise to go slowly at first, adding one or two new foods at a time and gradually working up to eating something fermented with every meal. If you are currently taking antibiotics or have a long history of using them, or are experiencing uncomfortable symptoms regularly such as gas, bloating, or diarrhea, or recurrent infections or allergies, you might benefit from taking a quality commercial probiotic supplement as well.

SEVEN WAYS TO ENJOY MORE FERMENTED FOODS

1. Eat some *naturally fermented vegetables* each day—raw sauerkraut, kimchi, curtido, dill pickles, pickle relish, capers, and the like. Make your own or seek out artisanal commercial brands prepared without vinegar, which are generally sold in the refrigerated section of natural food stores. There are so many ways to enjoy them—as condiments, in recipes, in sandwiches, with eggs, in salads, with meat, with nut butter on toast, or garnishing soup. Start with one-half teaspoon and work up to a tablespoon or two with each meal.

2. *Fermented dairy products* are a time-honored way to consume probiotics. Yogurt, kefir, and aged cheeses such as Parmesan and cheddar are concentrated sources of beneficial bacteria (Huffnagle and Wernick 2007), and fermentation reduces or eliminates hard-to-digest lactose. Beware of commercially sweetened yogurt, as it can contain very large amounts of sugar, more than ice cream in some cases. Enjoy yogurt alone, in smoothies, soups, and sauces, and as a condiment.

3. *Crème fraîche:* buy it or, better yet, make your own with the recipe in chapter 3. Use it as you would sour cream, enjoying its

mild flavor, or whip it to use on desserts. Or try making cultured ice cream using half crème fraîche and half buttermilk, sweetening it with maple syrup and whatever fruit is in season, and freezing it according to the directions for your ice-cream maker.

4. What do you do with the rest of the carton of *buttermilk* after you make crème fraîche? My grandmother used to drink buttermilk plain and marinate chicken in it, but I prefer it in pancakes, waffles, and muffins, mixing it with the flour the night before cooking or baking to soak overnight, neutralizing the phytic acid in the grains and rendering them more digestible and nutritious. While most commercially available buttermilk is pasteurized, it is still valuable for its acid and metabiotic content.

5. *Drink your ferments.* A small glass of kombucha, Beet Kvass (chapter 2), Rosemary Lemonade, Hibiscus and Rose Hip Soda (both in chapter 3) or other lactofermented beverages with each meal will provide valuable enzymes and aid digestion. Or try starting the day with a cultured dairy smoothie, made from kefir or yogurt.

6. Eat *fermented animal products.* Did you know that salami and other traditional sausages are made by allowing lactic acid bacteria to ferment meat and spices? Seek out naturally cured meats without added nitrates for probiotic and metabiotic benefits. Another useful item is fermented fish sauce. I use this to give salt, umami, and fermented enzyme power to curries, stir-fries, soups, and many Asian dishes. Fish sauce doesn't taste fishy when used in small quantities, just flavorful. Another choice for flavor power is salt-cured anchovies.

7. *Miso,* the fermented paste made from beans and/or grains, provides probiotics and phenols for a healthy gut. Enjoy miso soup; try chickpea miso in your next batch of pesto; blend miso into creamy soups, salad dressings, and sauces; and use it as a shortcut stock or alternative to bone broth. Be sure not to boil soups after adding miso, as this will kill some of the live bacteria.

Autumn Recipes

Cooking in the autumn is a joy, as you draw on the abundance of the harvest season. Spending a little more time in the kitchen now will help you slow down after summer's busyness and create the nourishing foods of fall, strengthening your immunity in preparation for the winter months. Strive for a balance of pungent and sour flavors to support your body's adjustment to the cooler weather.

Autumn Shopping List

Animal Products: pastured beef, lamb, pork, and goat; sustainable, seasonal fish and seafood; wild game; pastured and/or raw dairy products; lard, ghee, and other animal fats

Grains: wheat, rye, brown basmati and long-grain brown rice

Vegetables: corn, shelling beans, artichokes, winter squash, sweet potatoes, leeks, green beans, shallots, onions, cabbage, olives, wild mushrooms, Jerusalem artichokes, rutabagas, fennel, snap peas, turnips, beets, celery root, celery, carrots, parsnips, Brussels sprouts, green garlic, radishes, cauliflower, chile, watercress, spinach, bok choy, broccoli

Fruits: grapes, pears, Asian pears, raspberries, chestnuts, blackberries, quince, persimmons, strawberries, apples, pomegranates, kiwis, mandarins

Nuts: walnuts, almonds, hazelnuts, pecans

Herbs, Spices, and Condiments: cilantro, mint, parsley, and other fresh herbs; apple cider vinegar; umeboshi plum vinegar; raw sauerkraut; kimchi and other fermented vegetables; tamari, miso, and shoyu; fermented fish sauce

Pickled Beets and Turnips

These pickles are a gorgeous deep red, and they're a wonderful way to increase your intake of ultranourishing beets. They can accompany many savory dishes or get tossed into salads.

Makes 1 quart

3 medium beets, trimmed and scrubbed but not peeled (about 1 pound)

1 bunch small turnips, quartered and sliced thin (about 1 cup)

½ red onion, sliced thin

½ teaspoon mustard seeds

1 tablespoon sea salt

Preheat the oven to 400°F.

Put the beets into a baking dish and roast until tender when pricked with a fork, 45 minutes to 1 hour. Let cool; then quarter and slice thinly. Combine all the ingredients in a bowl and let sit at room temperature for 6 or more hours, until the vegetables begin to exude some liquid.

Pack the vegetables and their liquid, salt, and mustard seed into a clean widemouthed 1-quart mason jar and press down until the liquid rises above the top of the vegetables. If there is not enough liquid to cover the vegetables, add ½ teaspoon more salt dissolved in a couple of tablespoons of filtered water. Find a smaller jar or bottle that will fit inside the mason jar, and use it to press the vegetables down below the level of the liquid. Cover the whole thing with a tea towel secured with a rubber band, place the jar on a saucer to catch any drips, and allow it to ferment at room temperature.

Check daily to be sure the vegetables stay submerged, and taste to see how the flavor is developing. They'll get increasingly sour each day, and the flavor becomes more complex over time, eventually becoming less pleasant. When the pickles have achieved a flavor that pleases you (typically after fermenting for 3 days to 2 weeks), remove the inner jar, seal with a lid, and store in the refrigerator. The pickles will keep for many months.

Curtido

Curtido is an immunity-enhancing condiment common throughout Central America in various forms. Similar to sauerkraut, it tastes great with dishes with a New World flavor profile. Try it with scrambled eggs and black beans for breakfast.

Makes 1 quart

1 head green cabbage, sliced thinly

1 small red onion, sliced

2 or 3 carrots, scrubbed but not peeled, grated

1 bunch red radishes, thinly sliced or left whole if they are really small

1 teaspoon sea salt

2 jalapeños, quartered lengthwise, seeded, and sliced thinly

2 teaspoons chopped fresh oregano leaves, or ½ teaspoon dried Mexican oregano

Place the cabbage, onion, carrots, and radishes in a large bowl. Add the salt and massage the vegetables with your clean hands, squeezing and tossing them until they begin to release their liquid. Add the jalapeños and oregano and mix to distribute. Pack the mixture tightly into a widemouthed 1-quart mason jar, pushing down the vegetables until the liquid rises above the level of the cabbage. Put a smaller jar inside the mouth of the jar to keep the curtido submerged. Cover with a clean tea towel and secure with a rubber band. Leave out at room temperature for 3 to 5 days or more, tasting each day until it is sour enough for you. Then fasten the lid on the jar and store it in the fridge. The curtido will keep for months.

Bok Choy and Butternut Kimchi

This is a simplified version of kimchi, the popular Korean condiment. It makes a great side dish and complements most foods with an Asian flavor profile, such as Five Spice Short Ribs (chapter 5).

Makes about 1 quart

2 cups coarsely chopped bok choy

1 bunch red radishes, sliced in half

1 cup peeled butternut squash, chopped into ½-inch pieces

3 tablespoons sea salt

4 cups water

2 stalks green garlic, coarsely chopped

6 dried Thai chiles, or 1 teaspoon dried chili flakes

One 1- to 2-inch knob fresh unpeeled gingerroot, sliced

½ small red onion, sliced

½ teaspoon fermented fish sauce

Combine the bok choy, radishes, and squash in a large bowl. In a separate container, dissolve the salt in the water and pour this brine over the vegetables. Place a plate that's a little smaller than the bowl over the vegetables to keep them submerged, and allow them to soften for several hours to overnight.

The next day, drain the vegetables, reserving the brine. Make a spice paste by finely chopping the garlic, chiles, ginger, and onions, either by hand or in a food processor, and combining with the fish sauce. Mix the spice paste into the vegetables, and stuff it all into a widemouthed 1-quart mason jar. Press the vegetables down until the liquid rises above the level of the vegetables; add some of the reserved brine if necessary to cover the vegetables. Weight the vegetables down with a smaller jar or bottle and cover the whole thing with a tea towel secured with a rubber band. Allow to ferment for 5 to 8 days or more, tasting each day and ensuring that the vegetables stay covered with liquid. When it has fermented to your liking, secure a lid on the jar and store it in the refrigerator, where the kimchi will keep indefinitely.

White Bean–Kabocha Stew
with Herb Pesto

This dish is quite flexible, and can incorporate almost any seasonal vegetable. It also freezes well. Kabocha squash shines here, but other winter squashes, such as butternut and red kuri, are also delicious. It is wonderful topped with Herb Pesto (chapter 2) made with arugula and sage, but you can use a fruity olive oil as a garnish as well.

Makes 4 to 6 servings

1 cup dried great northern, baby lima, or other white beans

One 4-inch piece kombu

1 onion, coarsely chopped

1 carrot, scrubbed but not peeled, and coarsely chopped

1 stalk celery, coarsely chopped

1 bay leaf

3 tablespoons Ghee (page 52), rendered Duck Fat (page 116), or olive oil

1 cup coarsely chopped leek, both white and green parts

2 cups 1½-inch-cubed kabocha squash

1 quart filtered water, Savory Vegetable Broth (page 139), or Poultry Stock (page 115)

½ cup coarsely chopped celery leaves

2 teaspoons sea salt

Pepper

1 cup green beans, trimmed

2 pinches saffron, crumbled (optional)

Umeboshi plum vinegar

Herb Pesto (page 53)

The night before you plan to cook, soak the beans in water to cover by 2 inches. Alternatively, start a few days earlier and sprout the beans according to the directions in chapter 2.

When you're ready to cook, drain the beans and put them into a medium saucepan with the kombu, bay leaf, carrot, celery, and onion. Cover with water by 2 inches. Bring to a boil, reduce the heat to a simmer, and simmer until the beans are tender, for about 1 to 1½ hours. Drain the beans, reserving the cooking liquid, and remove and discard the bay leaf and kombu.

Using a large soup pot over medium heat, heat the fat. Add the leeks and sauté until they begin to turn golden, for 3 to 5 minutes. Pour in the water or stock and bring it to a boil over high heat. Add the squash, celery leaves, salt, and a few grindings of black pepper; reduce the heat; cover; and simmer for 20 minutes, until the squash begins to soften. Add the green beans, the white beans with their cooking liquid, and the saffron. Simmer for 15 minutes or until all ingredients are tender. Check the seasoning, adding salt, pepper, or plum vinegar as needed. Serve topped with herb pesto.

Roasted Root Vegetables

Roasted vegetables aren't so much a dish as a way of cooking and eating. They can be eaten topped with a fried egg for breakfast, in a salad or soup for lunch, and with virtually any entrée at dinner. Any time you turn the oven on in fall or winter, consider adding a tray of vegetables to roast as well—there is no doubt they'll get eaten. Roasting brings out a surprising sweetness in the pungent vegetables of fall, such as turnips and celery root; it makes a lovely complement to the richness of orange colored winter squash or yams. Adding herbs to the oil helps protect it from oxidative damage in the heat of the oven.

Makes 4 to 6 servings

2 tablespoons olive oil, melted Duck Fat (page 116), lard, or Ghee (page 52)

½ teaspoon sea salt

½ teaspoon dried rosemary or thyme

3 small turnips, rutabagas, daikon (white or pink varieties), potatoes, peeled celery roots, or a combination, cut into ¾-inch cubes (about 3 cups)

1½ cups ¾-inch-cubed winter squash, sweet potatoes, carrots, or a combination, peeled if desired (see note)

1 fennel bulb, cored and sliced into ¾-inch-thick diagonal slices (optional)

Preheat the oven to 450°F.

Put the olive oil or other fat into a small bowl and stir in the salt. Crumble the rosemary or thyme into the bowl with your fingers and stir to combine. Put all the prepped vegetables in a large bowl and toss with the seasoned fat until thoroughly coated. Spread the vegetables in a single layer on a rimmed baking sheet or large roasting pan, place it on the top rack of the oven, and roast for at least 20 minutes. Remove the vegetables, which should be starting to brown and become fragrant, and use a spatula to mix them. Return them to the oven and roast until tender when pricked with a fork and browned to your liking.

Note: The peels of all winter squash and root vegetables are both edible and nutritious, but the fibrous texture of some of them may not appeal to all tastes.

Duck Three Ways

Preparing a duck is a wonderful way to get comfortable working with whole animals. From one or two ducks you can have two great meals for two or a feast for four, plus stock and home-rendered fat for cooking. Take the time to scout out a source of sustainably raised duck in your area, and ask your butcher to cut it up for you, saving the fat separately.

Duck Breast with Balsamic Pomegranate Sauce

Serves 2 to 4

2 duck breasts

¼ teaspoon sea salt

Pepper

½ cup balsamic vinegar

½ cup pomegranate juice

Rub the breasts all over with the salt and sprinkle with pepper. If your butcher hasn't done so already, score the skin side of the breasts all over with a sharp knife, cutting through the skin but not into the flesh, about 1 inch apart.

In a small saucepan, combine the balsamic vinegar and pomegranate juice over medium heat. Bring to a boil and reduce the heat to low. Simmer until reduced by two-thirds and beginning to thicken, 15 to 20 minutes. Watch carefully in the last few minutes so that the sauce does not burn. Set aside.

Heat a heavy skillet over medium heat. Place the breasts, skin side down, in the skillet. After 5 minutes, pour off most of the hot fat and reserve for another use (as in braising the duck legs, see the next page); then continue cooking the breasts until deeply browned on the skin side, for a total cooking time of about 8 to 10 minutes. Turn the breasts over and sauté them in the hot fat for another few minutes. You'll be able to tell when the meat is done when it feels firm when pressed with your finger. Remove it from the pan and allow to rest on a plate for a few minutes.

To serve, slice it on the diagonal into ¼-inch slices and drizzle with the sauce. I like to serve additional sauce on the side for dipping, or you can serve the rest as a dip for seasonal fruit for dessert.

Braised Duck Legs with White Beans

Serves 2 or 3

Duck legs can be tough unless cooked slowly. Combining them with beans stretches their relatively small amount of meat, making a substantial dish for two or three people.

1 cup dried flageolet or cannellini beans

One 6-inch strip kombu

2 tablespoons Ghee (page 52), lard, olive oil, or Duck Fat (see previous page or page 116)

2 duck legs

1 small onion, sliced

2 carrots or parsnips, scrubbed but not peeled, diced

2 stalks celery, diced

2 bay leaves

Sea salt

Pepper

2 cups Poultry Stock (page 115), Savory Vegetable Broth (page 139), Bone Broth (page 138), or white wine

Chopped parsley for garnish

Soak the beans overnight in water to cover. In the morning, drain the beans, put them in a medium saucepan, and cover by 1 inch with cool water. Bring them to a boil, add the kombu, cover, turn the heat down to low, and allow to simmer while you prepare the duck.

Meanwhile, using a large skillet with a lid, heat the fat over medium heat. Brown the duck legs in the hot fat on both sides, for about 6 to 8 minutes per side. Move the duck to a plate and add the onion to the pan, sautéing it until it begins to turn golden, for 5 to 10 minutes. Add the carrots or parsnips, celery, and bay leaves, and sauté for a few minutes more, until the vegetables begin to release their fragrance. Add the browned duck legs back to the pan and season with salt and pepper. Add the stock or wine. Drain the beans and add them to the pan as well; then cover it and simmer everything together over low heat for 1½ to 2 hours, until the meat and beans are very tender. Serve garnished with chopped parsley.

Poultry Stock

Stock making can be as simple as simmering bones in water with a splash of vinegar. For those who prefer more precision, this recipe yields a very nourishing, gelatinous stock. This recipe calls for a single duck or chicken carcass, but feel free to save bones in your freezer until you have enough for a larger batch. Meat markets and specialty markets often carry chicken feet by the pound; they are worth seeking out as they will add a great deal of body and flavor to the stock.

Makes 8 to 10 cups, depending on the size of your pot

1 roasted chicken carcass, meat removed, or the bones from preparing a duck, as above

Giblets from the bird, if you have them, except the liver (see note)

8 ounces chicken feet (optional)

2 tablespoons apple cider or other mild vinegar

Place the carcass, giblets, and chicken feet in a slow cooker or large soup pot and cover with filtered water. Add the vinegar and let stand for at least 30 minutes. If you are using a slow cooker, turn it to high and allow the stock to come to a simmer. Then turn the heat down to low and let the broth cook for 8 to 24 hours. If you are using the stove top, bring the stock to a boil, cover, turn the heat down very low, and simmer for 8 to 24 hours. Turn off the heat and allow the stock to cool. Strain the stock and discard or compost the solids. Stock will keep for several days in the fridge and several months if frozen. Freezing some of your stock in ice cube trays and then storing them in a bag (be sure to label it!) in the freezer will give you a handy source of nourishing flavor to add to many dishes.

Note: Poultry liver will add a strong taste to the stock. If you have the liver, sauté it up with onions, chop it finely, and enjoy it on buttered toast for a cook's vitamin-rich treat.

Duck Fat

If you got a packet of duck fat along with your duck, you can render it at home. Duck fat is especially wonderful for roasting potatoes, or use it in the duck dishes in this chapter. To render, simply chop finely as much duck skin and fat as you can find, either by hand or in a food processor. Put the skin and fat in a pot with a heavy bottom and simmer on medium heat until the fat is completely liquefied and clear, and the skin is brown and crisp. Be careful not to burn the fat. Take the pot off the heat, cool, and strain. The fat will keep in the refrigerator for several months and will freeze indefinitely. The browned bits of skin are delicious eaten as is, or as a salad garnish with a bit of salt.

Paper-Wrapped Fish

Choosing fish and seafood gets ever more complex, as the human impact on their habitat grows daily. Yet these foods are superbly nutritious. Eating a variety of sustainably sourced fish and seafood allows you to balance environmental and nutritional concerns. This way of preparing fish is very simple and gives great results with most fillets and whole, cleaned fish you might find at your local famers' or fish market. Seek out unbleached parchment paper at a gourmet or natural market. I have found that for many recipes, including this one, preheating the oven is not really necessary and that skipping this step can save fuel; if you do so, be mindful that the food will take rather longer to cook.

Makes 2 to 4 servings

1 **pound seasonal, sustainably sourced fish fillet or whole fish, such as trout or sole**

2 **tablespoons butter**

1 **tablespoon chopped fresh herbs, such as fennel tops, cilantro, parsley, or thyme**

1 **organic lemon**

Sea salt

Pepper

Preheat the oven to 350°F. If using filleted fish, cut or portion it into two pieces, each about ½-inch thick. Lay out 2 pieces of foil, and cover with 2 pieces of parchment paper slightly smaller than the foil. If using whole fish, lay out foil and paper as above for each fish.

Dot the fish with butter and sprinkle with herbs. Slice the lemon in ¼-inch-thick rounds and remove the seeds. Distribute the lemon slices over the fish, or inside the body cavity if using a whole fish. Wrap up each portion first in the parchment and then in the foil, crimping the edges to seal tightly.

Place the foil packets on a rimmed baking sheet and bake for 20 to 30 minutes. You can check for doneness by opening a packet and inserting the blade of a small, sharp knife into the fish's flesh. If the flesh is opaque, it's done.

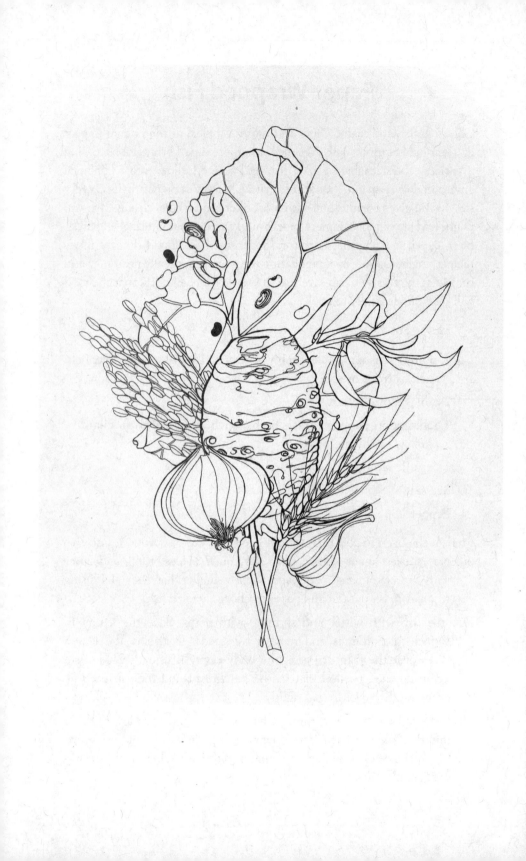

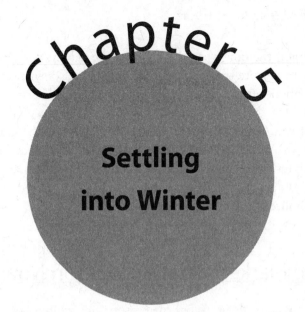

Chapter 5

Settling into Winter

During the winter months, all things in nature wither, hide,
return home, and enter a resting period...this is a time when yin
dominates yang. Therefore one should refrain from overusing
yang energy. Retire early and get up with the sunrise, which is
later in winter. Desires and mental activity should be kept quiet
and subdued.

The Yellow Emperor's Classic of Medicine (Ni 1995, 6)

Ah, winter. It seems to really hit only after the holidays, when the long
nights of January march on and the credit card bills come due. The classics teach us to consolidate our energy in the winter, becoming more inter-
nally focused and quieter, talking less and listening more. It is a great time
to cook more, too, creating long-simmered soups and stews, braising,
roasting, and baking to warm both the house and the body.

Winter is the time when the energy of the kidneys predominates, and it is wise to nurture these organs. The kidneys not only govern filtration and urination but are, in the Asian tradition, considered the root and foundation of the body's energy, determining your overall health, the health of your bones, your reproductive capacity, and the grace (or lack thereof) with which you age. This chapter will reconnect you to traditional winter foods and cooking methods, and remind you to take the respite and deep nourishment that are too often neglected and that can truly revitalize you in this season of rest.

At the Market: What's in Season Now

For humans throughout history, merely surviving winters has been a challenge, in part because fresh food is scarce. The three (or more, depending on where you live) months of winter still present a challenge to those of us seeking to eat locally. As the modern supermarket knows no seasons, it is possible to eat your way through winter without changing your diet at all, but that would not be wise. A stroll through the farmers' market, if you have one that operates year-round in your area, will remind you of the warming foods the body thrives on now: storage vegetables, like carrots, parsnips, celery root, onions, winter squash, yams, and potatoes; and the sturdy greens that taste best in cold weather, such as kale and collard greens. The fruits of the season include apples and pears from cold storage; kiwi fruit; oranges, lemons, grapefruits, kumquats, and other citrus fruit; and dried fruit. While tropical and out-of-season fruit appears at the supermarket shipped in from the Southern hemisphere, it is best avoided, as such fruit tends to overcool the body and to lose nutrition in its shipping and storage. Winter is the time to dig deep into the freezer and pantry and eat up the last of summer's harvest you squirreled away, to cook up dried grains and beans, and to enjoy more of that winter staple, sustainably sourced meat. The energy of the plant world is in storage in roots, seeds, and tubers, and your diet should reflect this, incorporating more of these foods, in the form of grains, beans, nuts, and seeds, than you eat in warmer seasons, and minimizing your intake of cold and raw foods, except for raw fermented foods like pickles.

Cooking Styles for Deep Nourishment

Cooking styles for winter should be long; think roasting, stewing, braising, baking. While long cooking times reduce the content of certain vitamins, they also make minerals more available to the body, especially in bone broths and stocks. Longer cooking brings out nutrients and qualities in foods that attune our bodies to the energy of winter. Make a soup, a stew, and then a soup again. Winter is the most appropriate time of year to consume some fried foods, as well. Most important is your choice of fat in which to fry. Animal fats, which are highly saturated, can be heated to high temperatures with little damage, creating nongreasy fried foods. Choose lard, bacon grease, duck fat, or ghee for pan- or deep-frying. Less saturated vegetable oils typically don't perform well at high heats, but peanut oil is one of the most stable. While heated oils can be hard to digest, this type of cooking is very warming, providing stamina in winter. Complement fried foods with fermented foods, as is done in many cultures to support digestion, for example, the pairing of Japanese tempura with pickled daikon radish.

THE FLAVORS OF WINTER

As the nights lengthen into winter, eating more salty food will help consolidate your energy, turning your focus inward. But not all salt is created equal. Truly unrefined salt, such as Celtic sea salt, and salt mined from ancient sea beds, such as Real Salt, are not bright white but off-white or light pink, indicating the presence of the wide array of minerals naturally present in seawater. Using this type of salt, as well as eating traditional foods made with sea salt, such as miso, naturally fermented tamari or shoyu (traditionally brewed, high quality soy sauces), and pickles, supplies your body with important trace minerals. Refined salt is pure sodium chloride, stripped of the other minerals, and is much harder for the body to balance than natural salt. Remember that the chemical composition of our bodies is quite similar to seawater. Every good cook knows that adding the right amount of salt is crucial to achieving peak flavor in a dish. Seeking out bitter flavored foods, especially bitter, sturdy cooking greens like collards and turnip greens, also helps to consolidate energy within the body in winter time.

There is another flavor that can be associated with the water element, which intuitive cooks the world over seek to impart to food: *umami*. Umami, a deep, savory taste, was acknowledged scientifically in 1985 (Lehrer 2007) as the fifth flavor detectable by the tongue, quite distinct from sweet, sour, salt, and bitter. Umami is recognized as having the ability to balance tastes, round out the flavor of a dish, and impart a mouth-watering feeling to the tongue (Beauchamp 2009). The umami taste is imparted by the presence of L-glutamate, an amino acid that is released by cooking, aging, and fermentation. Foods that are high in umami include fish, shellfish, cured meats; fermented and aged products in general, such as cheeses, miso, and tamari; and certain vegetables and fruits, including asparagus, mushrooms, ripe tomatoes, cabbage, and spinach.

Traditional cuisines worldwide employ the umami flavor in everything from fish sauce, a traditional condiment or ingredient of every fish-eating culture (of which catsup is a feeble imitation, although it, too, is high in umami), to the use of broths and stocks in cooking. When you deglaze the pan in making a sauce, you are imparting umami flavors from the denatured proteins created by browning meats. The taste for umami is ingrained from birth, as human breast milk is high in umami. It has been argued that since umami signals the presence of protein, the taste for it is adaptive, meaning it guides us to eat foods that are important for health. Umami may also signal the presence of fermentation, which is also adaptive, since eating fermented foods is so beneficial. While the use of umami makes food taste better at any time of year, the rich flavors and longer, more complex cooking techniques of winter tend to liberate amino acids in foods and bring out the umami flavors in a dish.

The Kidneys in Chinese Medicine

In addition to their function of regulating urination, the kidneys in the Chinese medical system are also said to govern metabolism, reproduction, development, and longevity. They rule the lower back and knees, as well as sexual and certain hormonal functions. They provide energy and warmth for the body, paralleling the Western understanding of the function of the adrenal glands, located on top of the kidney organs. The kidneys govern maturation, development, and the aging process, right down to when we get gray hair. Signs of kidney imbalance include: fatigue; bone problems (especially the knees); low back, teeth, and ear problems; receding gums; hair loss; urinary and prostate issues; impotence; either too much or too little sex drive; excessive fear and insecurity; and bags or dark circles under the eyes. Your kidney energy can become depleted through overwork; chronic stress; long-term illness; insomnia or simple lack of sleep; drug use, particularly of stimulants; chemical exposure; excessive ejaculation or childbearing; and eating too much sweet food. To replenish depleted kidneys, you need rest and nourishment.

Traditional Foods to Strengthen the Kidneys

- Whole Grains: millet, wild rice, dark-colored varieties of grains, such as quinoa

- Vegetables: parsley, sea vegetables, yams

- Fruits: berries, especially dark berries; dried fruit

- Nuts and Seeds: almonds, black sesame seeds, walnuts

- Beans: all beans, particularly dark varieties such as black and kidney beans

- Animal Foods: bone broths, clams, crab, lobster, oysters, organ meats, pork

Dark-colored foods have a special affinity for the kidneys, which is likely due to their high content of *anthocyanins* and other powerful phytochemicals in their pigments. Seek out black sesame seeds; black rice, quinoa, and beans; and dark berries, such as blue- and blackberries, when in season. The kidneylike shape of dried beans reminds us of their affinity for these organs. Dark-colored beans are higher in antioxidants than most fruits, plus they are inexpensive and high in fiber. Soaking, sprouting, and cooking with kombu and spices are all important ways to increase the digestibility and nutrient content of beans.

Organ meats, especially liver and kidney, are nutritionally potent. They have been prized by traditional peoples throughout history, often more than the muscle meat mostly eaten today (Fallon 2000). Incorporating organ meats into your diet is well worth adjusting your palate for. Be sure to seek out organ meats from organic or pastured animals, as the quality of the organs directly reflects the health of the animal. Calf liver may be readily available at supermarkets and is a good choice because it is harvested while the animals are generally still grass-fed. Organic chicken liver may also be easy to find at natural food markets. If you are a novice regarding organ meats, start out with high-quality artisanal pâté or liverwurst to acquaint yourself with the rich flavor of liver. Then you'll be ready to try some liver or kidney recipes at home, such as the Chicken Liver Mousse (later in this chapter). See the resources section for cookbooks covering organ meats cookery in more depth.

The kidney energy governs the fundamental forms of yin and yang in the body. If your kidney yang, your deepest internal fire, is weakened, you may feel cold easily or have cold extremities, as well as experience low back and knee pain, impotence or infertility, frequent urination, low libido, edema, or asthma. Kidney fire naturally declines with age, and in China most people begin taking kidney-strengthening foods and herbs around midlife. Animal foods are particularly strengthening to the yang, and if your yang is very weak, it is very helpful to eat one to three servings of animal foods a day from organic, pastured, or wild animals.

TRADITIONAL FOODS TO STRENGTHEN KIDNEY YANG

- Whole Grains: oats, spelt, sweet brown rice, quinoa

- Vegetables: cabbage, garlic, kale, leeks, mustard greens, onions, parsnips, parsley, green onions, winter squash

- Fruits: cherries, dates, raspberries (use dried or frozen when not in season)

- Spices and Herbs: anise, black pepper, cinnamon, cloves, caraway, citrus peel, cumin, dill, fenugreek, fennel, ginger, rosemary

- Beans: adzuki and black beans

- Animal Foods: chicken, crab, lamb, lobster, organ meats, shrimp, trout, wild salmon

If your kidney yin, which functions like an internal coolant, gets depleted, you may experience a dry mouth and throat and mild sensations of heat, such as feeling warm or thirsty in the afternoon or evening, or night sweats. Dizziness, ringing in the ears, low back pain, menstrual irregularities, agitation, irritation, nervousness, insecurity and fear, excessive sex drive, and premature ejaculation are other symptoms of kidney yin deficiency. If your kidney yin needs strengthening, focus on rest and replenishment. Consuming at least one meal of the day in a watery medium such as soup will support your yin. High-quality sleep is the best natural tonic for your yin, so ensure that you get enough of it. You should avoid consuming too many warming spices, excessive exercise and sweating, and stimulants.

TRADITIONAL FOODS FOR NOURISHING KIDNEY YIN

- Whole Grains: amaranth, barley, millet, rice, wheat

- Vegetables: asparagus, beets, eggplant, potatoes, sea vegetables

- Fruits: apples, berries, lemon, grapes, mulberries, melon (in season)

- Beans: all dried beans, miso

- Animal Foods: anchovies, cultured dairy products such as yogurt and kefir, duck, goat cheese, raw cheese, eggs, organ meats, pork, shellfish, sardines

An even more esoteric, yet fundamental, aspect of the kidney energy, which is closely linked to the kidney yin, is the kidneys' function of storing the *jing*. Jing is said to be inherited from your parents, and it is your deepest essence, akin to the energy savings account of the body. The quality and quantity of your jing determines your health, life span, and aging process. Your daily energy is drawn from the air you breathe and the food you eat and, when these are insufficient for your needs, from your reserves of jing. Jing is depleted by stress, fear, overwork, worry, excessive ejaculation or childbearing, toxin exposure, and too much sugar in the diet. Jing cannot be replaced, but it can be enhanced through meditation; through the

Chinese exercise regimens of *tai qi* and *qi gong*, and yoga; and by eating certain tonic foods, many of which are very nutritive and high in essential fatty acids and vitamins B12, A, and D. The closest analog in Western physiology to the jing is our DNA, the code for life itself, which is stored in each cell and, like the jing, is subject to degradation over time.

Foods that can nourish the jing include the microalgae, chlorella, spirulina, and blue-green algae; barley grass and wheatgrass; fish and shell-fish; liver; cod liver oil; kidneys; bones and marrow and the broth made from them; almonds; raw milk and cheese; ghee; nettles; bee pollen; and *goji* berries (Chinese wolfberries). You'll find many of these foods in natural food markets. Choose only high-quality, organic or pastured substances to truly strengthen your jing.

Integrative Perspectives on Kidney Energy

Gum disease and tooth decay are almost universal among humans eating an industrialized diet, and these symptoms reflect widespread weakness in kidney energy among modern people. Bone problems, including *osteoporosis* and *osteoarthritis*, are widespread in the aging population (Cordain et al. 2005) and are also turning up more frequently in younger people. While most people think of our bones as a relatively inert, static tissue, in fact they undergo a constant process of breakdown and repair, and they function as the body's most significant reserves of minerals. For years, holistic nutritionists have counseled on the importance of balancing acid- and alkaline-forming foods in the diet, and this concept has finally begun to be recognized in mainstream nutrition as an important influence on health in general and the health of our bones in particular.

Acid and Alkaline: Another Yin and Yang

Because life on earth evolved in the ocean, our metabolic processes function best when our bodies are in the same slightly alkaline state as the ocean (Brown 2000). Your body's pH is tightly controlled; indeed, this is one of the homeostatic mechanisms that form the basis of health. The kidney organs assist in regulating the acid-alkaline balance in the blood through excreting urine of variable pH. If the blood becomes overly acid, the body must draw on its mineral reserves, particularly those in the bones, to buffer the acid and maintain homeostasis.

The food you eat influences the acid load of the body once it is metabolized. In general, alcohol, sugar, fats and oils, protein foods, and grains tend to acidify the body; dairy products and beans are more neutral and act as buffers; and fruits, vegetables (especially sea vegetables), and other mineral-rich foods, such as sea salt and miso, are alkalizing (Colbin 2009). While the typical Western diet, heavily reliant on grains, factory-farmed meat, and sweeteners, and low in minerals, tends to create a state of chronic, low-grade acidity, the diet on which humans evolved created a slightly alkaline state. A recent survey of contemporary research showed many benefits of a slightly alkaline diet: preventing and treating osteoporosis, age-related muscle wasting, calcium kidney stones, hypertension, and exercise-induced asthma, as well as slowing down age- and disease-related kidney damage (Cordain et al. 2005). It is notable that all of these health problems are connected to kidney function in the Chinese medical sense. It seems that our kidneys function best when the diet is slightly alkaline.

There are many ways to achieve a diet that is alkalizing. For most of us, simply maintaining a steady intake of vegetables and fruit will help bring us into balance. Since both meat and grains are acidifying, diets high in both will tend to be unbalancing. Combining beans and grains with vegetables and a lower intake of animal products is one pattern that can work well, while a higher intake of animal foods complemented by vegetables and some fruit works much better for other constitutions and climates. Including mineral-rich, highly alkalizing foods such as fermented foods made with sea salt, seaweed, and bone broths offers a simple way to shift your diet toward a more alkalizing one.

MINERALIZING YOUR DIET

One of the consequences of modern, industrial agriculture is that soil minerals have been consistently removed from the soils, often being washed into the sea through soil erosion. The ocean is a reservoir of minerals, so it is important to include foods from the sea in the diet regularly. Sea salt, fish and seafood, and sea vegetables provide an incredible diversity of minerals. Just as it is important to choose fish and seafood from sustainable fisheries and seek species low in contaminants, sourcing sea vegetables that are sustainably harvested from clean environments is very important, particularly because of the known ability of these plants to take up harmful compounds such as radioactive and industrial pollutants. Better yet, a well-planned seaweed foraging trip can stock your pantry for the year.

Most traditional diets that have had access to foods from the sea have included sea vegetables, including those of Japan, Korea, China, Iceland, Ireland, Scotland, Wales, Denmark, the Pacific Islands, and coastal North America. Sea vegetables are nutritional powerhouses, high in iron and calcium, and containing B vitamins, vitamin A, potassium, magnesium, phosphorus, iodine, and trace minerals like selenium, zinc, copper, and molybdenum. Sea vegetables are high in fiber, support water metabolism and elimination, and alkalize the body. The brown seaweeds, including *kombu, wakame, arame,* and *hijiki,* contain *alginic acid,* which binds and helps expel heavy metals and radioisotopes. Used for thousands of years in Chinese medicine, sea vegetables are said to soften hardness and promote urination, and are used in this and other traditional healing systems to treat goiter, cysts, hernia, edema, urinary tract infections, high cholesterol, high blood pressure, asthma, menstrual and menopausal symptoms, and more.

Sea vegetables are also one of the few sources of wild foods in many people's diets, offering nutrition that is simply unavailable in cultivated foods. They are nutrient dense and practically calorie free, the opposite of so many modern foods. They provide many of the nutrients available from fish and seafood, notably iodine and calcium, but are more sustainable. Strive to include them in your diet daily. Seaweeds can concentrate toxins from the waters in which they are grown, so know your sources! These are the major types of sea vegetables and some ideas for uses:

- Strand Seaweeds: arame, hijiki, sea palm—soak and use in salads, veggie dishes, soups

- Strip Seaweeds: kombu, wakame—add to soups and broths, or briefly soak and cut into strands and use as strand seaweeds, above

- Sheet Seaweeds: prepared and wild nori, dulse—toast or fry for toppings or sandwiches (lettuce, tomato, and dulse sandwich, anyone?), soups, and scrambles; use nori as a sushi wrapper

- Kombu: cook this flavor enhancer with all grains or beans for enhanced digestibility and nutrition, plus shorter cooking times for dried beans

- Seaweed as a Snack: crumble toasted nori, sea palm, or dulse with toasted nuts, or add to trail mix, or try Asian flavored nori sheets

Aging with Grace

In recent years, science has brought an intense focus to the study of the aging process, which is ruled by the kidneys in Chinese physiology. Two dominant theories of the science of aging describe it as a process of both oxidation and *caramelization,* an interaction between sugars and protein (Weil 2005). Both of these are strongly influenced by diet. Oxidation is likely the more familiar term of the two, and it is simply the chemists' term for the removal of electrons from ions or molecules. Refer to chapter 4 for a discussion of oxidation and nutritional strategies for protecting yourself against oxidative stress.

What about caramelization? Yes, it is the same process you employ in cooking when you caramelize onions, for example, an interaction between sugar and protein exposed to heat that produces browning and lovely umami flavors in food. These reactions happen in our bodies all the time, but they are accelerated if our blood sugar gets too high. Many longevity researchers today believe that the degeneration of aging is partially the result of the slow browning and caramelization of our tissues. Andrew Weil's work suggests that eating in a way that supports steady moderate blood sugar may be a useful long-term way to prevent diabetes, weight gain, heart disease, and many other chronic disorders that can cause illness and shorten the life span (ibid.). This echoes the warning of the *Nei Jing,* which advised over two thousand years ago that too much sweet food can harm the kidneys, weaken the bones, and cause the hair to fall out.

129

Threat to the Jing: Genetically Modified Organisms in the Food Supply

Over the last twenty years, changes have occurred in the natural world beyond anything our ancestors could have imagined. The most significant of these is the newfound ability of humans to alter the genetic code—the foundation of life, analogous to the kidney jing itself. This new type of genetic manipulation is utterly different from the selective breeding that has been practiced through the millennia and that produced most of humanity's food crops and animals and many of our medicinal herbs. Biotechnology enables scientists to insert genes from one species into another species—a process that can never happen in nature—creating *genetically modified organisms* (GMOs). New organisms thus created are frequently released into (or escape into) the environment, and have been known to make their way into wild and nongenetically modified populations. Once released, these *transgenic* organisms have an unpredictable life of their own—and they can never be recalled.

There are many reasons to be concerned about the risks of transgenic manipulation. The majority of transgenic crops are grown and eaten in the United States, making Americans the unwitting subjects of "one of the largest uncontrolled experiments in modern history" (Kimbrell 2007, 18). In a 2003 survey of Americans by ABC News, 93 percent supported the labeling of genetically engineered foods (Singer and Mason 2006), which is done in many countries, including the EU, Russia, China, Korea, Japan, Thailand, Australia, and New Zealand. Most multinational food corporations have two lines of products, those containing GMOs for the US and Canadian markets, and GMO-free products for other countries. Despite years of activists' efforts, Congress has yet to mandate GMO labeling. Instead, up to 75 percent of processed foods in supermarkets and restaurants in our nation contain genetically engineered ingredients, and approximately 60 percent of the corn, 89 percent of the soy, 83 percent of the cotton, and 75 percent of the canola grown in the United States is genetically engineered (Smith 2007).

How did these foods become so pervasive without public knowledge? It would seem logical that before a novel entity is introduced into the food supply, it should be tested for safety in animal and human feeding studies. Instead, the USDA and FDA, which share responsibility for the safety of the food supply, have relied on the concept of "substantial equivalence," simply assuming that transgenic foods are the same as naturally bred foods. The result is that most of these products have not been thoroughly tested (Shiva 2000). A survey of the animal feeding studies that have been done on genetically engineered foods reveals a myriad of potential threats to health. In the study that to date is widely considered the "the best designed and carefully controlled study of its type" (Smith 2007, 22), Arnad Pusztai, senior scientist at the prestigious British Rowett Institute, and a team of twenty researchers found that after both 10 and 110 day periods of eating GMO potatoes, young rats had damage to almost every organ system as well as abnormal proliferative cell growth in their stomachs and intestines (Ewen and Pusztai 1999; Smith 2007). The drama that unfolded after Pusztai met with the press and discussed his concern over the damage to the young rats is typical of the history of GMO foods. The potatoes were approved anyway, Pusztai was fired, causing an outcry among the scientific community, and it was later revealed that the Rowett Institute had received £140,000 in funding from Monsanto (Shiva 2000).

The vast majority of GMOs grown in the United States have been designed to do one or both of the following: to express resistance to a particular pesticide (such as Roundup or glyphosate, which is marketed by the company that makes the altered seed); or to continuously produce large amounts of *Bacillus thuringensis* or Bt toxin, a natural bacterial toxin also used by organic farmers to control weeds. In a study done by Monsanto in 2002, rats were fed their MON 863 Bt corn for ninety days and showed statistically significant changes, including increased basophils, lymphocytes, and white blood cells; reduced kidney weight; decreased reticulocytes (indicating a risk of anemia); and increased blood sugar (Hammond et al. 2006). The study methodology was widely criticized, and scientists worldwide called for follow-up on the findings; this was never done (Smith 2007). Despite these concerns, the corn was approved, and is now planted and consumed around the world. According to Monsanto's website, this strain of corn, MON 863, has different nutritional properties than the parent strain, containing less protein and vitamins and more carbohydrate.

Early safety assessments of genetically engineered foods assumed that transgenic material would not survive digestion. However, more recent studies have confirmed that transgenes and gene fragments *can* and *do* survive digestive processes (Smith 2007). In the only study of human feeding on GMO foods conducted to date, seven volunteers who'd had previous ileostomies (surgical procedures that bring a portion of the small intestine to the skin surface) were fed a soy burger and soy milkshake made of Monsanto's Roundup Ready soybeans. Three of the subjects were later found to have the soy transgenes in their gut bacteria (Netherwood et al. 2004). Interestingly, the researchers inferred that the gene transfer had taken place prior to the study intervention, and suggested that the likelihood of gene transfer is dependent on repeated exposure. As most Americans are eating GMOs daily, it is likely that transgenes are being widely expressed in their gut flora. This is particularly disturbing in light of all the contemporary research that highlights the importance of gut bacteria and its complex effects on health (Guarner and Malagelada 2003). Consider that all transgenes contain not only the trait, such as pesticide resistance, that was intentionally inserted, but also use antibiotic-resistant genes as markers. It's reasonable to hypothesize that this could lead to the spread of antibiotic resistance among humans. This was the basis of Britain's rejection of one strain of transgenic corn (Shiva 2000). A 2011 study looking at pesticides associated with GMOs that the manufacturer claimed are broken down in digestion found them present in the majority of women, both pregnant and nonpregnant, and their fetuses (Aris and Leblanc 2011), a finding that has frightening implications for the health of future generations.

The story of Starlink corn highlights another category of health risks posed by GMO foods, as well as the major environmental threat of genetic contamination. Starlink is a GMO corn variety manufactured by Aventis that was approved for animal feed only, not human consumption, because of the risk of increased allergenic potential. The GMO variety was planted on less than 0.5 percent of the acreage planted of corn in the United States, but it quickly contaminated the entire food supply. In 2000, the discovery of Starlink corn in taco shells after several people experienced severe allergic reactions sparked a recall of three hundred corn products and cost Aventis $150 million in the cleanup effort (Cummings 2008). There were 115 documented cases of transgenic contamination between 1999 and 2005, in which unapproved GMOs were found or approved GMOs were found where they don't belong, such as in the fields of certified organic farmers. The Union of Concerned scientists reported in 2004 that the conventional seed supply is now "pervasively contaminated" with transgenes. The risk of transgene transmission from transgenic crops to conventional crops to weedy relatives of crop plants to wild plants is very real (Gurian-Sherman 2006). Genetically engineered plantings have, in fact, *never* been shown to increase yields and have widely resulted in increased use of pesticides, as well as inducing pesticide resistance (Gurian-Sherman 2009; Shiva 2000).

Healthy people depend on healthy ecosystems, and diversity is one of the basic principles of ecological health. Genetic engineering of food crops promotes—in fact depends upon—the suppression of diversity (ibid.). Environmental damage from GMOs has already occurred and will certainly continue if they continue to be planted where genetically altered genes can contaminate other plants (which is, functionally, nearly anywhere). All of us striving for optimal health and the health of our planet must act to protect the planetary ecosystem from the enormous threat posed by human manipulation of the genetic code. Author and GMO researcher Jeffrey Smith estimates, based on the European experience, that if 5 percent of American consumers began to consistently reject GMO foods, the food industry would act quickly to remove them from the food supply (Smith 2007). Where do you start? In your kitchen, of course.

KEEPING A GMO-FREE KITCHEN

1. Choose organic food. Certified, 100 percent organic food is the only packaged food that is, by definition, GMO free. If food is simply labeled "organic," it may contain up to 30 percent non-organic ingredients, which are liable to contain GMOs. Most other packaged food, especially any food containing soy, corn, cottonseed oil, sugar beets, canola, or their many derivatives, is likely to contain GMOs. At this writing, a GMO-derived artificial sweetener called neotame has been approved and is allowed in organic foods without being listed on the label. For the latest information on this fast-changing topic, contact the food advocacy organizations listed in the resources section.

2. Read the PLU (price lookup) labels on produce—the little stickers on individual apples, for instance. If the PLU is four digits, the food was grown conventionally and may or may not

be a GMO. If it is five digits, and the first digit is "9," it's organic; if the first digit of five is "8," the food is a GMO.

3. Grow or forage for your own food. When choosing seeds, be sure to choose organic and heirloom varieties, as the majority of seed companies are now owned by Monsanto. Learn to save seeds and develop your own seed bank of GMO-free seeds. Share seeds through a local seed library.

4. Be wary with dairy. Many conventional farmers inject cows with a genetically modified growth hormone, rBGH, to boost production. To avoid this hormone, which is damaging to the health of dairy cows and may be linked to increased cancer rates (O'Brien and Kranz 2009), choose certified organic dairy or dairy products labeled "rBGH-free" or "rBST-free." As this book goes to press, Congress has approved the planting of GMO alfalfa, which may eventually contaminate the entire alfalfa crop of the United States, the major source of forage for dairy cows. Keep abreast of the status of GMO alfalfa through one of the organizations listed in the resources section.

5. Ask your local markets and restaurants to go GMO free, or at least label food that may contain GMOs. Visit http.responsibletechnology.org for tips on working with retailers and for a downloadable non-GMO shopping guide.

6. See the resources section for contact information for organizations working on GMOs and other food safety issues.

Winter Recipes

In winter, dig deep into your pantry and create hearty dishes that warm and nourish your body to the core, featuring the produce that stores well or can be harvested this season.

Winter Shopping List

Animal Products: beef, pork, chicken, goat, shellfish, organ meats, nitrate-free preserved meats

Beans: all dried beans, especially adzuki and black beans

Grains: barley, rice, millet, oats, dark varieties of grains such as rice and quinoa

Vegetables: Brussels sprouts, cabbage, celery root, collard greens, endive, escarole, kale, kohlrabi, leeks, onions, parsnips, radishes, ruta-bagas, sea vegetables, turnips, winter squash

Fruits: lemons, oranges, kumquats, grapefruits, and other citrus; kiwi; dried fruit

Herbs, Spices, and Condiments: ginger, sea salt, miso, tamari, pickled vegetables

Chicken Liver Mousse

It can be a challenge to find organic or pastured chicken livers, but it is worth the effort, as the condition of the internal organs directly reflects the health of the animals. Grating whole nutmeg fresh with a box grater or Microplane adds a whole dimension of flavor beyond that of preground nutmeg. Serve this dish as a first course or part of a picnic lunch with sourdough bread, crackers, or crudités for dipping.

Makes about 1 cup

12 ounces pastured or organic chicken livers

4 tablespoons unsalted butter

1 shallot, finely chopped

2 cloves garlic, finely chopped

¼ cup brandy

¼ teaspoon freshly grated nutmeg

1 teaspoon fresh herbs such as thyme and tarragon, or ½ teaspoon dried herbs

Sea salt

Freshly ground pepper

3 to 4 tablespoons Crème Fraîche (page 51)

Trim any tough membranes or white tendons from the chicken livers. Using a heavy-bottomed sauté pan, heat the butter over medium heat. Add the chopped shallot and garlic, and cook and stir until the shallot is soft, 5 or 6 minutes. Add the chicken livers to the pan and cook, stirring gently, until they begin to brown but are still a bit soft, about 6 minutes. Add the brandy and herbs, turn the heat up to medium-high, and cook until most of the liquid has evaporated, 3 to 4 minutes more. Remove from heat and allow to cool slightly.

Transfer the livers to the bowl of a food processor fitted with the blade attachment. Add the nutmeg, a few grindings of pepper, a pinch of salt, and the crème fraîche, and process until you have a very smooth paste. Taste and correct the seasoning if needed. Pack the mousse into

2 half-pint mason jars or other similar containers. Refrigerate until the mousse begins to firm up a bit, which will take several hours. Bring to room temperature before serving.

Bone Broth

Broth making is a traditional way to get the most flavor and nutrition from an animal carcass. Not only is bone broth highly mineralizing and alkalizing, it also works to heal the lining of the intestinal tract and strengthen digestion. The long cooking extracts maximum nutrition from the bones. You can purchase bones from your butcher, a farmers' market, or a meat CSA, or simply save bones from meals in your freezer. When you have enough to fill your stockpot or slow cooker one-half to two-thirds full of bones, make broth; use it right away or freeze it for future meals. Freezing some stock in ice cube trays makes it easy to enhance the flavor and nutrition of many a dish.

Makes about 4 quarts

1 pound or more of fresh, meaty bones such as oxtail or shank, or 1 quart or more leftover beef, lamb, or pork bones

1 tablespoon lard or bacon grease (if using fresh bones)

1 pound or more beef soup bones (marrowbones)

1 tablespoon apple cider vinegar

Filtered water

If you are using fresh bones, heat a cast-iron or other heavy skillet over medium-high heat. Add the fat and, when it is melted, add the bones, browning well on all sides; this will take about 20 minutes. Combine the browned bones with the soup bones and vinegar in a large stockpot or slow cooker, and add filtered water to cover. Bring to a boil, cover, and reduce the heat to a very slow simmer. Simmer for 36 to 48 hours.

If you are using leftover bones, combine them with the soup bones and vinegar, and filtered water to cover, in a large stockpot or slow cooker. Bring to a boil, cover, and reduce the heat to a very slow simmer. Simmer for 36 to 48 hours.

Allow the stock to cool, and strain before using in a recipe or freezing.

Savory Vegetable Broth

This broth has the nutritional potency and deep savory flavor of a well-made bone broth without animal ingredients. The secret is the use of roasted onions and garlic, and the addition of kombu, a source of umami and of diverse minerals. Another wonderful thing: you don't need to peel any of the vegetables, which saves a lot of time. You should rinse them before using, however. It is an excellent habit to set aside vegetable trimmings, such as the dark-green portions of leeks, winter squash seeds and strings, celery tops, and the like for use in stock, freezing until there are enough.

Makes about 6 quarts

2 onions, coarsely chopped

1 head garlic, sliced in half horizontally

1 teaspoon olive oil

1 big leek, trimmed and cut into thirds

1 bunch celery, including the heart and leaves, cut into thirds

3 yams or sweet potatoes, quartered

2 cups cubed winter squash of any type

Two 6-inch strips kombu

2 bay leaves

1 teaspoon sea salt

Preheat the oven to 450°F. Place the onions and garlic in a roasting pan and toss with the olive oil to coat. Roast until they are beginning to brown, about 20 minutes.

Put the onions and garlic with all of the other ingredients in a large stockpot, fill it with water to within 2 inches of the top, cover, and bring to a boil. Remove the lid and simmer on low heat for 2 hours. Strain and use, or allow to cool completely before transferring into smaller containers for freezing.

Five Spice Short Ribs

Braising on the bone with warming spices epitomizes winter meat preparation. You can use oxtail, lamb or beef shank, or similar on-the-bone meat cuts with this recipe to delicious effect. Go ahead and use water if you don't have any broth or stock on hand, but be sure to stash the leftover bones in your freezer for a future batch of Bone Broth (earlier in this chapter). Serve with rice and Bok Choy and Butternut Kimchi (chapter 4), alongside Roasted Root Vegetables (chapter 4), or with a simple purée of cauliflower.

Makes 3 or 4 servings

1 tablespoon pastured lard, bacon grease, Ghee (page 52), or olive oil

2 pounds beef short ribs

1 onion or large leek, diced

2 stalks celery, diced, or 3/4 cup diced celery root

2 carrots or parsnips, scrubbed and diced

3 cloves garlic, crushed, or 2 stalks green garlic, sliced

5 quarter-sized slices fresh gingerroot

½ teaspoon Chinese five spice powder

2 cups Bone Broth (page 138), Savory Vegetable Broth (page 139), or water

3 tablespoons tamari or fermented fish sauce, or a combination

1 tablespoon maple syrup

1 teaspoon rice vinegar

Zest and juice of 1 orange

Using a large, heavy pot such as a Dutch oven, heat the fat and brown the ribs on all sides; this will take at least 10 to 15 minutes. Add the onions, lower the heat to medium, and continue to cook and stir until the onions begin to soften, about 5 minutes. Stir in the celery, carrots, garlic, and ginger, and continue to sauté for 2 minutes. Add the five spice powder, broth, tamari, maple syrup, and vinegar, and bring to a boil. Cover the pot and reduce the heat to a simmer. Cook on low for 1 to 2 hours, until the meat is very tender and beginning to fall off of the bones.

Move the ribs to a plate, add the orange zest and juice to the sauce, and turn up the heat again to high to reduce the liquid, stirring occasionally, until the liquid reduces by a third and begins to thicken and turn glossy, about 10 to 15 minutes. Add the ribs back to the pot and heat thoroughly, and then serve with the sauce.

Two Oyster Stew

The two oysters used here are the bivalve and the mushroom. Combining these delights makes a luscious dish that strengthens the kidneys, lungs, and spleen, and that is full of beneficial fats, vitamins, minerals, and immune-stimulating polysaccharides.

Makes 2 or 3 servings

4 slices nitrate-free bacon

1 leek, white and pale green parts, diced

1 large carrot, diced

1 celery stalk, diced

½ fennel bulb, diced

2 bay leaves

8 ounces oyster mushrooms, bases trimmed and brushed free of any dirt

2 cups Bone Broth (page 138), Poultry Stock (page 115), Savory Vegetable Broth (page 139), or water

1 teaspoon fermented fish sauce

1 cup peeled, diced celery root or potatoes

½ cup white wine

One 10-ounce jar fresh, shucked oysters or 1 dozen fresh oysters, shucked, liquor reserved

2 tablespoons brandy (optional)

2 tablespoons minced parsley

¼ cup Crème Fraîche (page 51)

Sea salt

Freshly ground pepper

Juice of ½ lemon

Place the bacon in a heavy skillet, such as cast-iron, over medium heat. Fry the bacon, turning frequently, until it is browned but not yet crispy, and move to a plate. Pour off all but a thin layer of the bacon fat (save this in a jar for future use) and add the leeks. Sauté for a few minutes, until the leeks begin to soften; then add the carrot, celery, fennel, mushrooms, and bay leaf, sautéing for a few minutes more, until the vegetables begin to soften and release their aromas. Transfer the vegetables to a medium soup pot; add the bone broth, fish sauce, and celery root; cover; and bring to a simmer over low heat.

Return the skillet to medium heat, and add the wine to the pan to deglaze, using a spatula to scrape up the browned bits from the bottom of the pan into the wine. Scrape this into the soup.

Allow the soup to simmer until the vegetables are tender, around 15 minutes. Chop the bacon coarsely. Add the oysters and their liquor; the bacon; the brandy, if you are using it; and the parsley, and simmer for about 5 minutes, until the oysters are just tender. Remove the bay leaf. Turn off the heat and stir in the crème fraîche. If you would like a thicker soup, remove about a cup of the soup to a bowl and purée with a hand blender, or in a food processor or blender, until smooth. Stir this back into the soup, and season with salt, pepper, and lemon juice before serving.

Sesame Seaweed

This dish is popular even with seaweed neophytes. The sesame and sea-weed together pack a powerful punch of calcium, iron, and, of course, iodine.

Makes 2 to 4 servings

1 ounce sea palm, arame, or hijiki (about 1 cup loosely packed)

1 onion, sliced

1 tablespoon sesame or olive oil

2 tablespoons tahini

½ teaspoon tamari

Umeboshi plum vinegar

Soak the seaweed in cool water to cover for 10 to 15 minutes; then drain, saving the water for soup stock (or to add to bathwater to soften and nourish the skin, or use for fertilizer). Heat the oil in a skillet over medium heat and add the onion, sautéing until it begins to color, about 8 minutes. Add the seaweed and continue to sauté until the seaweed begins to get tender, about 5 to 10 minutes more, depending on the type. Stir in the tahini and a splash of water if the tahini is very thick. Keep stirring until the tahini is evenly distributed; then stir in the tamari until all is smooth. Finish with a dash (or so) of the vinegar to taste. Serve as a side dish, or use as a pastry or filo dough filling.

Variations

- Add carrots cut in matchsticks after the onions; use almond butter or peanut butter instead of tahini; add garlic with the onions; or use several tablespoons of whole toasted sesame, sunflower, or pumpkin seeds instead of or with the tahini.

Slow-Cooker Carnitas

A staple dish in my household year-round, this is an easy meal for a weeknight that will feed you many times more. The pork cooks in its own fat and juices in a slow cooker, maintaining a rich flavor without using quite as much precious lard as traditional preparations of carnitas. A single roast will yield many servings of tasty pork, which is great wrapped in tortillas with homemade guacamole and Curtido (chapter 4), served alongside beans and rice or on top of a bed of greens with salsa for a taco salad sans tortilla chips, or used to enrich a brothy soup of beans and vegetables.

Makes 10 or more servings

One 3-pound bone-in pork shoulder roast or Boston butt roast, preferably from a pastured animal

½ teaspoon sea salt

½ teaspoon ground cumin

½ teaspoon Mexican oregano

2 tablespoons pastured lard or bacon grease

2 or 3 dried hot chiles

1 onion, sliced

2 bay leaves

Chopped cilantro, for garnish

Rub the roast all over with the sea salt several hours or the night before you plan to cook it, cover, and refrigerate until you are ready to cook. Combine the cumin and oregano in a small bowl and rub this all over the roast. Heat the fat in a cast-iron or other heavy skillet over medium-high heat. Brown the roast thoroughly on all sides; this will take about 20 minutes. Place the chiles, onion, and bay leaves in the bottom of a slow cooker and turn on the heat. Add the roast and pour in any remaining fat from the bottom of the skillet. Cover and cook 4 to 6 hours on high or 8 to 10 hours on low heat, until the meat is utterly tender and falling apart. Before serving, turn off the heat, move the meat to a cutting board, discarding the seasonings, and shred it with two forks. Serve garnished with chopped cilantro.

Chocolate Truffles

Chocolate is a great gateway "drug" for getting other good things into people, like high-antioxidant dried fruits and nuts, immune-stimulating coconut oil, and even powdered adaptogenic herbs, such as maca or Siberian ginseng, which support the body in adapting to stress and act as kidney tonics. I've also made these truffles with carob powder instead of cocoa for my loved ones who don't indulge in chocolate.

Makes 2 cups

1 cup almonds, walnuts, pecans, or other nuts of your choice

½ cup raisins or prunes

¼ cup coconut oil

½ cup cocoa powder

1 tablespoon blackstrap molasses

1 teaspoon cinnamon

⅛ teaspoon cayenne pepper

Pinch of sea salt

½ teaspoon vanilla or almond extract

2 to 4 tablespoons powdered maca, Siberian ginseng, or other herbs (optional)

Soak the nuts overnight, or for several hours at least, in filtered water to cover. Add the raisins or prunes to the soaking nuts an hour or two before you plan to make the truffles.

Drain the nuts and fruit, and place them into a food processor. Grind into a paste, add the remaining ingredients, and blend until smooth. Roll into small balls, then coat with more cocoa powder. Store the truffles in the fridge for up to a month, and bring to room temperature for serving.

Almond Macaroons

Proving that cookies can also be nutrient-dense, these treats are not overly sweet, especially if you choose cocoa nibs over chocolate chips. The cinnamon helps keep your blood sugar stable, too. Seek out almonds at a farmers' market or farm stand to avoid those that have been chemically sterilized, or else look for steam-sterilized almonds at a natural food store.

Makes 2 dozen

2 large pastured egg whites

½ **cup organic evaporated cane juice, or coconut or palm sugar**

Pinch of sea salt

1 teaspoon cinnamon

Zest of 1 organic orange

⅛ **teaspoon cardamom**

3 cups sliced almonds

⅔ **cup Fair Trade chocolate chips or cocoa nibs**

Preheat the oven to 350°F.

In a mixing bowl, whisk the egg whites, sugar, and salt until well combined, and stir in the cinnamon, orange zest, and cardamom. Gently mix in the almonds and chocolate chips until they are evenly distributed in the batter. Line 2 baking sheets with parchment paper or silicone mats, or grease lightly with butter, and drop the batter by the tablespoon onto the sheets, forming it into flat mounds. Bake for about 15 minutes, until golden on top and dry on the bottom, and allow to cool before eating or storing, well-sealed, at room temperature for up to a week.

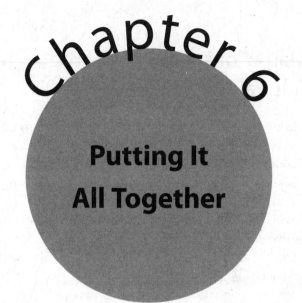

Chapter 6

Putting It All Together

The wheel of the year keeps turning: the sleeping seeds of winter awaken again as the sprouts and shoots of spring blossom into the fruits of summer and mature into the fullness of autumn, only to die back and sleep until spring returns. The rise and fall of seasonal energy is echoed in your body each day in your cycles of sleeping and waking, and over the span of your life, from birth through growth, maturation, and death. Attuning your diet to this cycle supports your health in many ways, by tying you more closely to the cycles of nature, bringing you the outstanding nutrition of fresh food and the pleasures of preparing it seasonally, and strengthening and cleansing each of your internal organs in turn through the year.

The Many Consequences of the Agricultural Transition

Chinese medicine is fundamentally an ecological medicine, concerned with restoring and maintaining the health of human beings in relation to their environment. Traditional Chinese nutrition can be seen as a system that teaches the healthiest way for people to eat *after* humans started farming. After all, humans evolved before agriculture. Human bodies evolved to run on a hunter-gatherer diet, and we turned to agriculture and animal husbandry only about ten thousand years ago. There is pervasive evidence that the transition to agriculture had a negative effect on human health (Diamond 1987).

Recently, an international group of researchers in human nutrition identified seven crucial nutritional changes from our ancestral preagricultural diets that are linked to the advent of chronic disease: 1) an increase in glycemic load; 2) a decrease in omega-3 and an increase in omega-6 fatty acid consumption; 3) an increase in the proportion of carbohydrates (primarily refined) combined with a reduction in protein intake; 4) a drop in micronutrient intake; 5) a shift in acid-base balance toward a chronic slightly acid, rather than alkaline, state; 6) a higher sodium-potassium ratio; and 7) a reduction in fiber intake (Cordain et al. 2005). Many of these changes arose from a shift in the diet toward a reliance on grains, particularly refined grains, and refined vegetable oils, concentrated sweeteners, and dairy products as major sources of calories.

Following the eating style and cooking techniques in this book will allow you to shift your diet closer to the healthy diet on which humanity evolved. You can decrease the glycemic load of your diet and improve macronutrient proportions by choosing whole instead of refined foods, incorporating healthy fats into your cooking, and harnessing the power of lactic acid fermentation and sprouting. By choosing healthy pastured animal fats, avoiding refined vegetable oils, eating sustainable fish and seafood and lots of leafy greens, you'll increase your omega-3 intake and decrease your omega-6. Simply eating seasonal produce, prepared to maximize digestion, will increase your intake of vitamins and minerals; doing this while avoiding refined salt and choosing sea salt and other mineral-rich foods such as seaweed will improve the sodium-potassium ratio of your diet. A whole foods diet provides plenty of fiber, and when you balance your intake of meats and grains with produce, you move toward a beneficial alkalizing diet.

Fine-Tuning Your Diet

You might find that entirely eliminating dairy and grains, or other foods that are recent entries into the human food supply, will bring you even greater health and energy than a diet that includes these foods. You can use the food journal introduced in chapter 1 now to reevaluate the effects of specific foods. If you identify a food to which you suspect you have an adverse response, try using the Spring Cleanse in chapter 2 as an elimination diet, avoiding the foods in question for several weeks before reintroducing one at a time, eating each food several times in one day and assessing your response. Food sensitivities often clear up after a few months of avoiding a particular food. If the issue is true *gluten intolerance*, a genetic condition that is linked to autoimmune disorders and a host of other maladies and that seems to be becoming more common, the best treatment is total avoidance of gluten for life (Brostoff and Gamlin 2000).

Transitioning to a seasonal diet of properly prepared whole foods will bring greater health and vitality to most people. If you have done this and have persistent low energy or otherwise suboptimal health, be sure to visit your health practitioner. A holistic nutritionist or acupuncturist trained in Chinese nutrition can also help you in tailoring your diet more closely to your individual health needs and constitution.

The Impact of Industrial Agriculture

In the past hundred years or so, humans have yet made another agricultural transition, from traditional agriculture to industrial agriculture. This transition has had grave consequences both to human health and the health of the planet. While US agriculture produces more calories per person than ever before (3,800 calories per person per day in 2000 according to USDA sources, almost twice what the population needs), this increase in production has actually led to a 5 to 40 percent loss of nutrients in foods over the last hundred years (Davis 2009). Most Americans are overfed and undernourished. The grossly energy-inefficient industrial food system takes a whopping ten calories of fossil-fuel energy to produce each calorie of food, and up to 37 percent of greenhouse gas production is from industrial agriculture (Pollan 2008).

While the rhythm of the seasons has always shaped human lives, in recent years it has become more and more obvious that human activities are shaping the climate and even altering the seasons, bringing warmer winters and earlier springs to most regions (Thomson 2009). Climate change is now in turn affecting agricultural yields. According to Stanford professor David Lobell, there has been about a 5 percent decline in production of corn and wheat worldwide (except in North America), along with a 6 percent rise in prices of these crucial foodstuffs over the past thirty years due to the changing climate (Lobell et al. 2011). Other research reported in the *New York Times* in June 2011 suggested that declining global harvests have been affected by adverse weather events, such as floods and hurricanes, linked to climate change (Gillis 2011). On the other hand, organic agriculture has been shown in numerous studies to actually promote carbon sequestration (Rodale 2011). Sourcing your food seasonally, organically, and locally is a significant way each of us can help address climate change, as is being mindful of our energy use in getting our food and in cooking it. While our individual acts are important, collective action is a must if we want to really transform the broken food system in North America and around the globe. Consider getting involved in one of the many groups that are tackling these difficult issues—I list several of my favorites in the resources section.

My hope is that as you've worked your way through this book you've been inspired to try new foods and cooking techniques and you have come closer to a steady diet of home-cooked, local, seasonal food. This takes a big commitment of time, energy, and money, but the profound benefits make it well worth the effort. Eventually, cooking and eating seasonally becomes a way of life, as it was for our grandmothers and our ancestors, and it will be a source of continuing vitality and great pleasure for ourselves and those we love—and may even help transform the world.

Ten Tips for Busy Cooks

1. Cook once, eat twice (or more). Cook a double batch of grains or beans, and the extras can go into the next meal or the freezer. When you turn on the oven, consider what else can go in to be cooked for a future meal—a whole squash, perhaps, or a batch of beets for salad or pickling. Many leftovers can become an unconventional breakfast or brown bag lunch.

2. Cook on Sunday for the week. A half day spent cooking a large pot of beans and a soup and beginning a fermentation project can be the start of several meals for later in the week. If you tire of eating the same dish, freeze (and label!) half your batch in single-serving containers instead.

3. Think ahead. It becomes automatic: while doing dinner dishes, I'm thinking about what we're having for breakfast. In the morning, I'm planning dinner. What needs to be soaked, sprouted, or defrosted for the next few meals?

4. Shop with a list. Obvious to some, a revelation to others, this is also a good way to stick to your budget.

5. Keep your pantry well stocked. Having grains and beans, oils, condiments, spices, dried fruit, and canned seafood on hand, combined with the stores in your freezer (see below), will prevent many a trip for take-out.

6. Make good use of your freezer (part 1). Instead of packaged "convenience foods," keep it filled with cooked beans, meat, leftover soups and stews, pesto, and broth, and you'll have the ingredients for a real meal at the ready. Frozen broth and beans defrost quickly on the

stove top while you chop and sauté whatever fresh vegetables are on hand to make a delicious soup or stew. Top with Sauerkraut, Crème Fraîche, or Herb Pesto (all in chapter 2) and you're dining on real food faster than it takes to heat up a TV dinner in the oven.

7. Make good use of your freezer (part 2). Save bones and vegetable trimmings for stock until you have enough to make up a batch. Freeze cooled, strained stock in mason jars, leaving plenty of headroom to prevent breakage, or in repurposed yogurt or other plastic food containers.

8. Become a food producer, not just a consumer. Gardening, sprouting, foraging, urban farming, and fermentation mean you always have real food close at hand.

9. You don't have to do it all yourself. Cook with friends or neighbors and share the results. Become an expert sauerkraut maker and trade your creations for your neighbor's famous preserves. Find or start a barter market. I trade my Chocolate Truffles (chapter 5) for a friend's homemade raw goat feta.

10. Make it automatic. Picking up my CSA produce box and meat and egg shares takes less time than a trip to the market, and the regular schedule makes having real food around the house easy. Like a gym membership, paying for food in advance helps ensure that it gets eaten. And the steady and ever-changing supply of produce inspires new recipes and adventures in fermentation, a great way to preserve any surplus from your CSA or garden.

Resources

Food Sources

To find farmers' markets and CSAs in your area:
www.localharvest.org

For a national directory of pasture-based farms:
www.eatwild.com

For producers of pastured meat:
www.americangrassfed.org

Advocacy Organizations

Slow Food USA
20 Jay Street, Suite M04
Brooklyn, NY 11201
Tel: 718-260-8000 or 877-SlowFoo(d)
www.slowfoodusa.org

Slow Food emerged as a counterpoint to the ubiquity of fast food, and is a global grassroots movement linking the pleasure of food to building community and sustainability.

Weston A. Price Foundation
PMB 106-380
4200 Wisconsin Avenue NW
Washington, DC 20016
Tel: 202-363-4394
www.westonaprice.org

The Weston A. Price Foundation disseminates the research of nutrition pioneer Dr. Weston Price and is dedicated to restoring nutrient-dense food to the food supply through education, research, and activism.

The Center for Food Safety
660 Pennsylvania Ave SE, #302
Washington, DC 20003
Tel: 202-547-9359
Fax: 202-547-9429
www.centerforfoodsafety.org

The Center for Food Safety works to protect human health and the environment by curbing the proliferation of harmful food production technologies such as genetic engineering and by promoting organic and sustainable agriculture.

Institute for Responsible Technology
PO Box 469
Fairfield, IA 52556
Tel: 641-209-1756
www.responsibletechnology.org

The Institute for Responsible Technology works internationally to educate the public and policy makers about genetically modifed foods and crops.

Reading

Cooking

Fallon, S. 2000. *Nourishing Traditions: The Cookbook That Challenges Politically Correct Nutrition and the Diet Dictocrats*. With Mary Enig. Warsaw, IN: NewTrends Publishing.

Can replace *The Joy of Cooking* on your cookbook shelf.

Fearnley-Whittingstall, H. 2007. *The River Cottage Meat Book*. Berkeley: Ten Speed Press.

The bible of sustainable meat cookery.

Katz, S. E. 2003. *Wild Fermentation: The Flavor, Nutrition, and Craft of Live-Culture Foods*. White River Junction, VT: Chelsea Green Publishing.

Started the fermentation revolution.

Prentice, J. 2006. *Full Moon Feast: Food and the Hunger for Connection*. White River Junction, VT: Chelsea Green Publishing.

Lyrically calls for a return to seasonal eating and cooking methods.

Growing Your Own Food

Carpenter, N. 2009. *Farm City: The Education of an Urban Farmer*. New York: Penguin Press.

A memoir of adventures and misadventures on the radical edge of urban farming.

Flores, H. C. 2006. *Food Not Lawns: How to Turn Your Yard into a Garden and Your Neighborhood into a Community*. White River Junction, VT: Chelsea Green Publishing.

The title says it all.

Kaplan, R., and K. R. Blume. 2011. *Urban Homesteading: Heirloom Skills for Sustainable Living.* New York: Skyhorse Publishing.

The most soulful of the current crop of homesteading books, firmly grounded in the principles of permaculture, an approach to designing communities and agricultural systems modeled on the relationships found in nature.

Ruppenthal, R. J. 2008. *Fresh Food from Small Spaces: The Square-Inch Gardener's Guide to Year-Round Growing, Fermenting, and Sprouting.* White River Junction, VT: Chelsea Green Publishing.

Straightforward guide to producing your own food, even in tiny spaces.

Nutrition

Haas, Elson M. 2006. *Staying Healthy with Nutrition: The Complete Guide to Diet and Nutritional Medicine.* Berkeley, CA: Celestial Arts.

The most helpful single resource on holistic nutrition.

Haas, Elson M. 2003. *Staying Healthy with the Seasons.* Berkeley, CA: Celestial Arts.

This edition updates a classic in integrative medicine, which first introduced traditional Chinese seasonal healing wisdom to the West.

References

Aaronson, P. I. and, J. P. T. Ward. 2007. *The Cardiovascular System at a Glance*. Malden, MA: Blackwell Publishing.

Allport, S. 2006. *The Queen of Fats: Why Omega-3S Were Removed from the Western Diet and What We Can Do to Replace Them*. Berkeley: University of California Press.

Aris, A., and S. Leblanc. 2011. Maternal and fetal exposure to pesticides associated to genetically modified foods in Eastern Townships of Quebec, Canada. *Reproductive Toxicology* 31 (4):528–33.

Baker, S. M. 2003. *Detoxification and Healing: The Key to Optimal Health*. Chicago Contemporary Books.

Beauchamp, G. K. 2009. Sensory and receptor responses to umami: An overview of pioneering work. *American Journal of Clinical Nutrition* 90 (3):723S–727S.

Benbrook, C:, et al. 2008. "New evidence confirms the nutritional superiority of plant-based organic foods." Accessed December 9, 2010. www .organic-center.org/science.nutri.php?action=view&#0022; report_id=126.

Bjelakovic, G., and C. Gluud. 2007. Surviving antioxidant supplements. *Journal of the National Cancer Institute* 99 (10):742–743.

Brostoff, J. and L. Gamlin. 2000. *Food Allergies and Food Intolerance: The Complete Guide to Their Identification and Treatment*. Rochester, VT: Healing Arts Press.

Brown, S. E. 2000. *Better Bones, Better Body: Beyond Estrogen and Calcium: A Comprehensive Self-Help Program for Preventing, Halting, and Overcoming Osteoporosis*. Los Angeles: Keats Publishing.

Campbell-McBride, N. 2007. *Put Your Heart in Your Mouth*. Cambridge: Medinform Publishing.

Carlsen, M. H., B. L. Halvorsen, et al. 2011. The total antioxidant content of more than 3100 foods, beverages, spices, herbs and supplements used worldwide. *Nutrition Journal* 9:3.

Castelli, W. P., J. T. Doyle, et al. 1977. HDL cholesterol and other lipids in coronary heart disease: The cooperative lipoprotein phenotyping study. *Circulation* 55 (5):767–72.

Chardigny, J. M., F. Destaillats, et al. 2008. Do trans fatty acids from industrially produced sources and from natural sources have the same effect on cardiovascular disease risk factors in healthy subjects? Results of the Trans Fatty Acids Collaboration (TRANSFACT) study. *American Journal of Clinical Nutrition* 87 (3):558–66.

Colbin, A. 2009. *Whole-Food Guide to Strong Bones: A Holistic Approach*. Oakland, Calif.: New Harbinger Publications.

Cordain, L., S. B. Eaton, et al. 2005. Origins and evolution of the Western diet: health implications for the 21st century. *American Journal of Clinical Nutrition* 81 (2):341–54.

Crawford, M., C. Galli, et al. 2000. Role of plant-derived omega-3 fatty acids in human nutrition. *Annals of Nutrition and Metabolism* 44 (5–6):263–65.

Cummings, C. H. 2008. *Uncertain Peril: Genetic Engineering and the Future Of Seeds*. Boston, MA.: Beacon Press.

Davis, D. R. 2009. Declining fruit and vegetable nutrient composition: What is the evidence? *HortScience* 44 (1):15–19.

Davis, D. R., M. D. Epp, et al. 2004. Changes in USDA food composition data for 43 garden crops, 1950 to 1999. *Journal of the American College of Nutrition* 23 (6):669–82.

Dethlefsen, L. and D. A. Relman. 2011. Incomplete recovery and individualized responses of the human distal gut microbiota to repeated antibiotic perturbation. *Proceedings of the National Academy of Sciences* 108 (Suppl 1):4554–61.

Diamond, J. 1987. "The worst mistake in the history of the human race." *Discover* May, 64–66.

Dragland, S., H. Senoo, et al. 2003. Several culinary and medicinal herbs are important sources of dietary antioxidants. *Journal of Nutrition* 133 (5):1286–90.

Duke, J. A. 1997. *The Green Pharmacy: New Discoveries in Herbal Remedies for Common Diseases and Conditions from the World's Foremost Authority On Healing Herbs.* Emmaus, PA: Rodale Press.

Erasmus, U. 2007. *Fats That Heal, Fats That Kill.* Summertown, TN: Alive Books.

Ewen, S. W., and A. Pusztai. 1999. Effect of diets containing genetically modified potatoes expressing Galanthus nivalis lectin on rat small intestine. *Lancet* 354 (9187):1353–4.

Fallon, S., P. and M. Enig. 2000. *Nourishing Traditions: The Cookbook That Challenges Politically Correct Nutrition and the Diet Dictocrats.* Warsaw, IN: New Trends Publishing.

FDA/USDA. 2003. "Listeria monocytogenes risk assessment." Accessed December 2, 2010. www.fda.gov/Food/ScienceResearch/Research Areas/RiskAssessmentSafetyAssessment/ucm183966.htm.

Flood, J. E., and B. J. Rolls. 2007. Soup preloads in a variety of forms reduce meal energy intake. *Appetite* 49 (3):626–34.

Fruehauf, H. 2011. "All disease comes from the heart." Accessed May 10, 2011. www.classicalchinesemedicine.org/2009/04/all-disease-comes-from-the-heart/

German, J. B., and C. J. Dillard. 2004. Saturated fats: What dietary intake? *American Journal of Clinical Nutrition* 80 (3):550–559.

Gillis, J. 2011. "A warming planet struggles to feed itself." *New York Times* June 5.

Golomb, B. A. 1998. Cholesterol and violence: is there a connection? *Annals of Internal Medicine* 128 (6):478–87.

Gross, L. S., L. Li, et al. 2004. Increased consumption of refined carbohydrates and the epidemic of type 2 diabetes in the United States: an ecologic assessment. *American Journal of Clinical Nutrition* 79 (5):774–9.

Guarner, F., and J. R. Malagelada. 2003. Gut flora in health and disease. *Lancet* 361 (9356):512–9.

Gurian-Sherman, D. 2006. "Contaminating the wild? Gene flow from experimental trials of genetically engineered crops to related wild plants." Washington, DC: Center for Food Safety.

———. 2009. "Failure to yield: evaluating the performance of genetically modified crops." Washington, DC: Center for Food Safety.

Guyton, A. C. 1991. *Textbook of Medical Physiology*. Philadelphia: Saunders.

Halweil, B. 2004. *Eat Here: Homegrown Pleasures in a Global Supermarket*. New York: Norton/Worldwatch.

Hammond, B., J. Lemen, et al. 2006. Results of a 90-day safety assurance study with rats fed grain from corn rootworm-protected corn. *Food and Chemical Toxicology* 44 (2):147–60.

Herron, R. E., and J. B. Fagan. 2002. Lipophil-mediated reduction of toxicants in humans: an evaluation of an ayurvedic detoxification procedure. *Alternative Therapies in Health and Medicine* 8 (5):40–51.

Ho, P. Y., and F. P. Lisowski. 1997. *A brief history of Chinese medicine*. Singapore; River Edge, NJ: World Scientific.

Hu, F. B., J. E. Manson, et al. 2001. Types of dietary fat and risk of coronary heart disease: A critical review. *Journal of the American College of Nutrition* 20 (1):5–19.

Huffnagle, G. B., and S. Wernick. 2007. *The Probiotics Revolution: The Definitive Guide to Safe, Natural Health Solutions Using Probiotic and Prebiotic Foods and Supplements*. New York: Bantam Books.

Jones, D. S., ed. 2005. *Textbook of Functional Medicine*. Gig Harbor, WA: Institute for Functional Medicine.

Kaptchuk, T. J. 2000. *The Web That Has No Weaver: Understanding Chinese Medicine*. Chicago, IL: Contemporary Books.

Kimbrell, A, 2007. *Your Right to Know: Genetic Engineering and the Secret Changes in Your Food*. San Rafael, CA: Earth Aware.

Kingsolver, B., S. L. Hopp, et al. 2007. *Animal, Vegetable, Miracle: A Year of Food Life.* New York: HarperCollins Publishers.

Lee, S., and A. Kader. 2000. Preharvest and postharvest factors influencing vitamin C content of horticultural crops. *Postharvest Biology and Technology* (20):201–220.

Lehrer, J. 2007. *Proust Was a Neuroscientist.* Boston: Houghton Mifflin.

Libby, P. 2002. Inflammation in atherosclerosis. *Nature* 420 (6917):868–74.

Libby, P., P. M. Ridker, et al. 2002. Inflammation and atherosclerosis. *Circulation* 105 (9):1135–43.

Lipski, E. 2005. *Digestive Wellness.* New York: McGraw-Hill.

———. 2010. Traditional non-Western diets. *Nutrition in Clinical Practice* 25 (6):585–93.

Lobell, D. B., W. Schlenker, et al. 2011. Climate trends and global crop production since 1980. *Science* 333 (6042):616–620; EPUB May 5.

Long, C., and T. Alterman. 2007. "Meet real free-range eggs." *Mother Earth News* October-November, www.motherearthnews.com/Real-Food/2007-10-01/Tests-Reveal-Healthier-Eggs.aspx

Maciocia, G. 1989. *The Foundations of Chinese Medicine: A Comprehensive Text for Acupuncturists and Herbalists.* Edinburgh, New York: Churchill Livingstone.

Maki, D. G. 2006. Don't eat the spinach: Controlling foodborne infectious disease. *New England Journal of Medicine* 355 (19):1952–1955.

Masterjohn, C. 2007. Bearers of the cross: Crucifers in the context of traditional diets and modern science. *Wise Traditions* 8 (2):34–45.

———. 2010. Precious yet perilous: Understanding the essential fatty acids. *Wise Traditions* 11 (3):18–33.

Mateljan, G. 2001. *The World's Healthiest Foods.* Seattle: GMF Publishing.

McKay, D. L., C. Y. Chen, et al. 2011. Hibiscus sabdariffa L. tea (tisane) lowers blood pressure in prehypertensive and mildly hypertensive adults. *Journal of Nutrition* 140 (2):298–303.

Miller, D. and A. Sarubin-Fragakis. 2008. *The Jungle Effect: A Doctor Discovers the Healthiest Diets from around the World—Why They Work and How to Bring Them Home.* New York: Collins.

Mokdad, A. H., B. A. Bowman, et al. 2001. The continuing epidemics of obesity and diabetes in the United States. *Journal of the American Medical Association* 286 (10):1195–1200.

Molin, G. 2001. Probiotics in foods not containing milk or milk constituents, with special reference to Lactobacillus plantarum 299v. *American Journal of Clinical Nutrition* 73 Suppl. (2):380S–85S.

Mollison, B. 1993. *The Permaculture Book of Ferment and Human Nutrition.* Tyalgum, Australia: Tagari Publications.

Murray, M. T., J. E. Pizzorno, et al. 2005. *The Encyclopedia of Healing Foods.* New York: Atria Books.

Netherwood, T., S. M. Martin-Orue, et al. 2004. Assessing the survival of transgenic plant DNA in the human gastrointestinal tract. *Nature Biotechnology* 22 (2):204–9.

Ni, M. 1995. *The Yellow Emperor's Classic of Medicine: A New Translation of the Neijing Suwen with Commentary.* Boston: Shambhala.

O'Brien, R. and R. Kranz. 2009. *The Unhealthy Truth: How Our Food Is Making Us Sick and What We Can Do about It.* New York: Broadway Books.

O'Hara, A. M., and F. Shanahan. 2006. The gut flora as a forgotten organ. *EMBO Reports* 7 (7):688–93.

Ohlgren, S. and J. Tomasulo. 2006. *The 28-Day Cleansing Program: The Proven Recipe System for Skin and Digestive Repair.* Longmont, CO: Genetic Press.

Olshansky, S. J., D. J. Passaro, et al. 2005. A potential decline in life expectancy in the United States in the 21st century. *New England Journal of Medicine* 352 (11):1138–45.

Packer, L. 1991. Protective role of vitamin E in biological systems. *American Journal of Clinical Nutrition* 53 (4) Suppl.: 1050S–1055S.

Pandrangi, S. and L. F. LaBorde. 2004. Retention of folate, carotenoids, and other quality characteristics in commercially packaged fresh spinach. *Journal of Food Science* 69 (9):C702–7.

Pearsall, P. 1998. *The Heart's Code: Tapping the Wisdom and Power of Our Heart Energy.* New York: Broadway Books.

Pitchford, P. 2002. *Healing with Whole Foods: Asian Traditions and Modern Nutrition.* Berkeley: North Atlantic Books.

Pollan, M. 2008. *In Defense of Food: An Eater's Manifesto.* New York: Penguin Press.

Prentice, J. 2006. *Full Moon Feast: Food and the Hunger for Connection.* White River Junction, UT: Chelsea Green Publishing.

Radek, M., and G. P. Savage. 2008. Oxalates in some Indian green leafy vegetables. *International Journal of Food Sciences and Nutrition* 59 (3):246–60.

Robinson, J. 2004. *Pasture Perfect.* Vashon, WA: Vashon Island Press.

Rodale, M. 2011. *Organic Manifesto: How Organic Farming Can Heal Our Planet, Feed the World, and Keep Us Safe.* Emmaus, PA: Rodale.

Rolls, B. J., E. A. Bell, et al. 1999. Water incorporated into a food but not served with a food decreases energy intake in lean women. *American Journal of Clinical Nutrition* 70 (4):448–55.

Rosamond, W. D., L. E. Chambless, et al. 1998. Trends in the incidence of myocardial infarction and in mortality due to coronary heart disease, 1987 to 1994. *New England Journal of Medicine* 339 (13):861–7.

Rosengren, A., S. Hawken, et al. 2004. Association of psychosocial risk factors with risk of acute myocardial infarction in 11119 cases and 13648 controls from 52 countries (the INTERHEART study): Case-control study. *Lancet* 364 (9438):953–62.

Sachs, J. S. 2007. *Good Germs, Bad Germs: Health and Survival in a Bacterial World.* New York: Hill and Wang.

Shiva, V. 2000. *Stolen Harvest: The Hijacking of the Global Food Supply.* Cambridge, MA: South End Press.

Simopoulos, A. P. 1998. Overview of evolutionary aspects of omega 3 fatty acids in the diet. *World Review of Nutrition and Dietetics* 83: –11.

Sinatra, S. T. 2005. *The Sinatra Solution: Metabolic Cardiology.* North Bergen, NJ: Basic Health Publications.

Singer, P., and J. Mason. 2006. *The Ethics of What We Eat: Why Our Food Choices Matter.* Emmaus, PA: Rodale.

Smith, J. M. 2007. *Genetic Roulette: The Documented Health Risks of Genetically Engineered Foods.* Fairfield, IA: Yes! Books.

Smith, J. S., F. Ameri, et al. 2008. Effect of marinades on the formation of heterocyclic amines in grilled beef steaks. *Journal of Food Science* 73 (6):T100–5.

Steinkraus, K. H. 1983. Lactic acid fermentation in the production of foods from vegetables, cereals and legumes. *Antonie Van Leeuwenhoek* 49 (3):337–48.

Svilaas, A., A. K. Sakhi, et al. 2004. Intakes of antioxidants in coffee, wine, and vegetables are correlated with plasma carotenoids in humans. *Journal of Nutrition* 134 (3):562–7.

Taubes, G. 2007. *Good Calories, Bad Calories: Challenging the Conventional Wisdom on Diet, Weight Control, and Disease.* New York: Knopf.

Thomson, D. J. 2009. Climate change: shifts in season. *Nature* 457 (7228):391–392.

Thornton, J. W., M. McCally, et al. 2002. Biomonitoring of industrial pollutants: health and policy implications of the chemical body burden. *Public Health Reports* 117 (4):315–23.

Tucker, K. L. 2001. Eat a variety of healthful foods: old advice with new support. *Nutrition Review* 59 (5):156–8.

Waser, M., K. B. Michels, et al. 2007. Inverse association of farm milk consumption with asthma and allergy in rural and suburban populations across Europe. *Clinical and Experimental Allergy* 37 (5):661–70.

Weil, A. 2005. *Healthy Aging: A Lifelong Guide to Your Physical and Spiritual Well-Being.* New York: Knopf.

Wunderlich, S. M., C. Feldman, et al. 2008. Nutritional quality of organic, conventional, and seasonally grown broccoli using vitamin C as a marker. *International Journal of Food Science and Nutrition* 59 (1):34–45.

Yusuf, S., S. Hawken, et al. 2004. Effect of potentially modifiable risk factors associated with myocardial infarction in 52 countries (the INTERHEART study): Case-control study. *Lancet* 364 (9438):937–52.

Nishanga Bliss, MSTCM, LAc, is a licensed acupuncturist, integrative nutritionist, and professor of Chinese medicine at the Acupuncture Integrative Medicine College in Berkeley, CA.

Foreword writer **Liz Lipski, PhD, CCN, CHN,** is board-certified in clinical and holistic nutrition and is director of doctoral studies and educational director at Hawthorn University. She is author of *Digestive Wellness* and *Digestive Wellness for Children.*

Index

A

acid-alkaline balance, 126–127
adrenocorticosteroids, 71
advocacy organizations, 155–156
aging process, 129
agriculture: impact of industrial, 151–152; nutritional changes caused by, 150
alcohol consumption, 78
alfalfa, 134
alginic acid, 128
alkalizing foods, 127
Allport, Susan, 72
Almond Macaroons, 147
amaranth family, 32–33
anchovies, lamb with, 61
Animal, Vegetable, Miracle (Kingsolver), 28
animal fats, 121
animal foods, 10–11; autumn, 94–95, 104; cleansing diet and, 43–44; fatty-acid ratio of, 76; fermented, 102; organ meats, 123–124; pasture-raised, 10, 29–30; raw consumption of, 66, 89; spring, 29–30, 47; summer, 82; winter, 135
anthocyanins, 123
anticuchos, 68
antioxidants, 72, 75, 78–79
arame, 128
artichokes, 29
Asian health systems, 3, 5. *See also* Chinese medicine
asparagus, 27, 29
autumn, 93–117; cooking styles for, 95–96; in five element theory, 93; flavors of, 96; foods associated with, 94–95; large intestine related to, 99; lungs related to, 96–99; recipes for, 103–117; shopping list for, 104
autumn recipes, 103–117; Bok Choy and Butternut Kimchi, 107; Braised Duck Legs, 113–114;

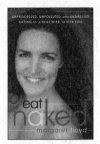
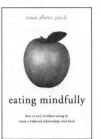
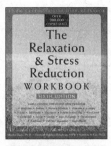
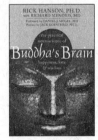
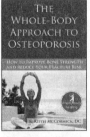
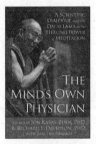